Home Care Nursing

An Orientation to Practice

Home Care Nursing

An Orientation to Practice

Carolyn J. Humphrey RN, MS
Assistant Professor
Nursing Program
Sacred Heart University
Fairfield, Connecticut

Paula Milone-Nuzzo, RN, PhD
Project Director/Research Scientist
Home Care Concentration
School of Nursing
Yale University
New Haven, Connecticut

APPLETON & LANGE
Norwalk, Connecticut/San Mateo, California

0-8385-3822-3

Notice: Our knowledge in clinical sciences is constantly changing. As new information becomes available, changes in treatment and in the use of drugs become necessary. The author(s) and the publisher of this volume have taken care to make certain that the doses of drugs and schedules of treatment are correct and compatible with the standards generally accepted at the time of publication. The reader is advised to consult carefully the instruction and information material included in the package insert of each drug or therapeutic agent before administration. This advice is especially important when using new or infrequently used drugs.

 Copyright © 1991 by Appleton & Lange
A Publishing Division of Prentice Hall

91 92 93 94 95 / 10 9 8 7 6 5 4 3 2 1

Prentice Hall International (UK) Limited, *London*
Prentice Hall of Australia Pty. Limited, *Sydney*
Prentice Hall Canada, Inc., *Toronto*
Prentice Hall Hispanoamericana, S.A., *Mexico*
Prentice Hall of India Private Limited, *New Delhi*
Prentice Hall of Japan, Inc., *Tokyo*
Simon & Schuster Asia Pte. Ltd., *Singapore*
Editora Prentice Hall do Brasil Ltda., *Rio de Janeiro*
Prentice Hall, *Englewood Cliffs, New Jersey*

Library of Congress Cataloging-in-Publication Data

Humphrey, Carolyn J., 1947–
    Home care nursing : an orientation to practice / Carolyn J. Humphrey, Paula Milone-Nuzzo.
        p. cm.
    ISBN 0-8385-3822-3
    1. Home care services—United States. 2. Home nursing—United States. I. Milone-Nuzzo, Paula. II. Title.
    [DNLM: 1. Home Care Services—United States. 2. Home Nursing—
United States. WY 115 H926h]
    RA973.H85 1991
    362.1′4′0973—dc20
    DNLM/DLC
    for Library of Congress   90-1058
                                                                CIP

Aquisitions Editor: Marion Kalstein-Welch
Production Editor: Sandra K. Huggard
Designer: Michael J. Kelly

PRINTED IN THE UNITED STATES OF AMERICA

To
Fred and Jonathan Gross and Joe, JohnPaul, and Jessica Nuzzo
Our community-based support systems

Contributors

The authors would like to thank the following colleagues
who contributed their expertise and support for this book.

Judith Benson, RN, BSN, MBA
Executive Director, Med Center Home Care
Danbury, Connecticut
*Judy, as an expert in the field of high-tech home care,
contributed that section to Chapter 7.*

Laura Cestari, RN, MSN
Nursing Supervisor, VNA of South Central
 Connecticut
New Haven, Connecticut
*Laura contributed her excellent work on stress in home
care nursing for Chapter 5.*

Gail Grammatica, RN-C, MS
Pediatric Clinical Nurse Specialist and Manager
Pediatric Home Care Program
VNS of Rochester and Monroe County, Inc.
Rochester, New York
*Gail wrote the section on pediatric home care based on
her education and experience in the field.*

Susan Westrick Killion, RN, MS, JD
Associate Professor, Southern Connecticut State
 University
Attorney at law
New Haven, Connecticut
*Susan contributed the material on legal considerations
relating to documentation found in Chapter 3 and all
of Chapter 6, Legal Aspects of Home Care Nursing
Practice.*

Ruth Knollmueller, RN, BSN, MPH
Assistant Director, VNA and Home Care, Inc.
Waterbury, Connecticut
*Ruth wrote the section on supervision, which is an
integral part of Chapter 5, Interpersonal Aspects of
Home Care Nursing.*

Lucinda Martin, RN, BSN
Nursing Supervisor/Coordinator, Regional Visiting
 Nurse Agency
North Haven, Connecticut
*Cindy used her high level of knowledge as well as her
day-to-day experiences to bring practical insight to
home care documentation, especially in the Medicare
section.*

Contents

Preface

WHY THIS BOOK IS NEEDED

Together, we have over 30 years of experience in home care nursing, as direct providers, supervisors, educators, and in administration. As a result of these experiences, it became apparent to us that home health agencies often lacked the time and resources necessary to develop and implement comprehensive, structured orientation programs for new nursing staff. Also, the responsibility of orientation was not always delegated specifically within the organization, and there was no central place where agency information was gathered for the new nurse to review and use as a reference in the future. This haphazard orientation process, used by many agencies, can start the new nurse off on the wrong foot and make a lasting negative impression of home care, the agency, and the work habits that are expected of the nurse in that position. With the current shortage of nurses, inadequate orientation programs can also lead to increased staff retention problems—since there are so many positions open to nurses, new staff members will not stay in a position or with an agency that appears to offer a negative work experience.

We also noted that when it came to the subject of education, agencies would focus on continuing education opportunities and inservice programs but missed laying the proper educational foundation for continued learning by offering faulty initial orientation programs. This lack of emphasis on initial teaching leads to frustrated nurses, disappointed managers, and administrators who are concerned about recruitment and retention issues and their relationship to costs and productivity.

This book is meant to lay the foundation for the clinical practice of home care nursing by providing a sound, educationally based–reality focused orientation program. The figure below depicts the nursing practice model upon which this book is based. Nurses come to home care with the skills and knowledge acquired from their basic nursing education and subsequent clinical experiences. Orientation is designed to be the beginning of the home care nurse's practice, which will continue to be developed through continuing education, in-service programs, and, perhaps, eventually through higher education since examination of nursing trends suggests that the role of the advanced practice nurse is developed through higher education.

In addition to our personal observations, there are several other reasons, which are outlined in this book, why a well-organized orientation program will have a positive impact on the home care nurse.

- The home care system is radically different from

Nursing Practice Model

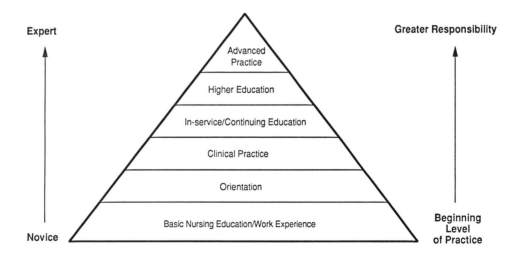

Educationally Based/Reality Focused

other areas of nursing practice. Independent decision making and clinical expertise relative to home care situations are essential for the nurse to be successful.

- Research supports the premise that the quality of orientation is directly related to work satisfaction, which leads to staff retention.
- State licensure, accreditation, and certification require that an appropriate orientation program be provided to home health agency staff. With the increasing emphasis on quality assurance issues, the quality of orientation programs will increase in importance.
- An effective orientation program can be cost efficient in two ways. First, the nurse is prepared to become a productive member of the organization in a short period of time, and, second, the well-prepared nurse has the potential to become a long-term productive employee who can assist in future recruitment and orientation of new staff.

WHAT THIS BOOK WILL DO FOR YOU

As educators and service providers, we have a background that has enabled us to develop an orientation program that is based on sound education principles while it stays focused on the real world of home care nursing practice. We believe that an orientation program is an educational experience for the new staff nurse and that the orientation process must include creative teaching strategies. The orientation program developed in this book is built upon teaching and learning principles and focuses on the clinical role specific to home care nurses. We have organized the book to provide the orientation coordinator with both creative teaching strategies and basic home care content that applies to all practitioners, regardless of the type of agency.

The downfall of most orientation programs is the focus on the **what** to be covered rather the **how**. It is not enough to give new nurses the policy and procedure manual to read and later discuss any questions they may have. We have set up a program that focuses both on the process of the orientation as well as the content.

INTENDED AUDIENCE

Home Care Nurse

The majority of information presented in this book is considered basic for any nurse working in home care today, regardless of the type of agency, specific nursing position, or client population served. Along with

the agency specific information addressed in the suggested orientation program and the personal assistance of the orientation coordinator, supervisor, and peers, this book provides the basic orientation and ongoing reference necessary for a professional nurse to become an effective home care practitioner.

It should **not** be assumed that if a nurse has worked in home care previously she has thorough knowledge of the many aspects of home care nursing practice that should be included in orientation. Too many times we have gone on visits with experienced nurses to find they do not know bag technique, how to contract with a client, timesaving hints to increase their productivity, and other information believed to be basic practice. This book is meant to be used by novice and experienced home care nurses with the material presented so that it relates to the specific agency. By using this book as a basis for orientation, the experienced nurse can put to practice what she already knows plus what she learns, and apply it to the new agency.

Orientation Coordinator or Supervisor

The term supervisor has been used throughout the book to denote the individual who is responsible for the home care nurse's orientation, and it can be used synonymously with any position in the agency that holds the ultimate responsibility for nursing orientation. This book provides the framework for a comprehensive orientation program that includes the basic material related to home care nursing combined with the addition of material specific to the individual home health agency.

This book is arranged in a format to encourage independent thinking, problem solving, and application of what has been learned to real-life patient and agency situations. The nurse being oriented is encouraged to review agency material that relates to information presented and to ask questions of various agency staff members to solidify her understanding. Also, case studies included throughout the text as well as questions at the end of each chapter provide the orientation coordinator with material needed to reinforce and evaluate learning. This evaluation can be in the form of written answers to the questions and small group or one-to-one conferences to discuss thoughts, feelings, and approaches to the practice applications presented.

The book is meant to be a workbook that can be used in initial orientation and for reference during the nurse's employment with the agency. It is suggested that the agency purchase one for each new nurse, allowing her not only to read it, but work out the exercises, make notes, and make it her own so it becomes the reference that will save both nurse and supervisor much time in her future work with the agency. The money spent initially for a sound orientation program using the book as guide and reference will be cost-effective for the agency since a productive nurse will be developed in a shorter period of time.

Student Nurse

Home care nursing material is increasingly being included in undergraduate and graduate curriculums in schools of nursing. Undergraduate students have clinical rotations in home health agencies where they are expected to utilize most of the information presented in this book. This reference can be especially useful in teaching R.N. to B.S.N. students the role and function of the home care nurse. Many graduate programs have tracks in home care, preparing their graduates for many specialty areas in the field.

This book is not meant to address advanced practice, but to provide a foundation for home care nursing practice that must be learned before mastery of the field can be approached. The authors, both educators as well as practitioners, have presented the material to be used by students as well as practicing nurses. The material and learning experiences can be used by teachers in the same way as is outlined for orientation coordinators. The material presented in this book has not been compiled in any other home care or community health nursing textbook and can, therefore, be a positive addition to class readings and required texts.

Acknowledgments

A book of this scope is only possible with the support and assistance of many people. We want to thank the following professional colleagues who have read sections of the manuscript and provided constructive feedback: Lazelle Benefield, Dee Coover, Judy Hays, Nancy Humiston, Virginia Humphrey, Donna Rozanski, and John Zak.

We also want to thank our colleagues from Sacred Heart University and Southern Connecticut State University for their assistance with this project.

Throughout the entire process of creating the orientation program and writing this book, Marion Kalstein-Welch, our editor, was a tremendous source of support and encouragement. She started as our editor and became our friend.

Our families, as always, have helped us by taking the kids, going to the grocery, and getting out of our way while we took over the kitchen table and the computer. Special thanks go to Pauline and John Milone, Jo-Anne Dora, Pamela Fornal, John Milone Jr., and to Josh, Marc, and Adam Gross.

Introduction

How to Use this Book

Each chapter begins with the objectives and key concepts covered in the chapter, as well as a list of the agency-specific materials needed to complete a stage of the orientation program. Before reading each chapter, the agency materials listed should be assembled for easy reference as the information is covered. At the end of each chapter are **Test Yourself** questions designed to allow the new staff nurse to review the content of the chapter and discuss the material learned with her supervisor or preceptor. This format is helpful to the nurse new to home care as well as the experienced home care nurse who is being oriented to a new agency.

Throughout the book the terms **client** and **patient** have been used synonymously to identify the individual recipient of care. **Family** and **significant other** have been used to describe the patient support systems with whom the home care nurse works to deliver care. The pronouns **her** and **she** have been used to refer to the home care nurse for convenience throughout the book. The terms **orientation coordinator** and **supervisor** have been used to identify the person(s) responsible for planning and implementing the home care nurse's orientation. **Home health agency** refers to any agency providing professional home care services, regardless of the type of agency, method of reimbursement, or geographical location. **Home** refers to the client's place of residence.

Chapter 1 gives an overview of the development and current status of the home care system in the United States. A discussion of the types of providers and staff working in a home health agency and their roles and functions give the new staff nurse a broad overview of the home care system and the personnel working in it. This chapter provides a framework for the remaining chapters, which are specific to home care nursing.

Chapter 2 begins with the definition of home care nursing and discusses the specific roles and functions of the home care nurse. The application of the nursing process to the home care setting is outlined, followed by a description of how to do a home visit with consideration given to universal precautions.

Chapter 3 discusses documentation of the nursing care provided, as it is an essential component of home care nursing practice. The general principles of home care documentation are covered as an introduction to how home care documentation differs from that in other practice areas. Documentation to satisfy Medicare regulations and how to write forms 485, 486, and 487 are also discussed in detail. An overview of the principles of quality assurance and how they relate to the agency and the nurse's practice are covered in the remainder of this chapter.

Chapter 4 details strategies for effective clinical management. Descriptions of case management, productivity issues, and contracting give the new staff nurse an understanding of how to use these strategies to become a more efficient and effective member of the staff. Since teaching is such an important intervention in home care, a detailed description of the development, implementation, and documentation of the teaching/learning process is included.

Chapter 5 addresses the interpersonal aspects of home care nursing practice with an extensive discussion of supervision—both how the home care nurse can supervise paraprofessionals and how she can work with her supervisor. Case studies are provided to facilitate an understanding of this important concept. The causes of stress in home care and strategies for dealing with stress on a daily basis are also included so the new nurse can prevent burnout.

Chapter 6 covers legal issues relevant to home care nursing practice. The first section, Basic Legal Considerations in Home Care Nursing, examines such legal considerations as confidentiality, witnessing documents, and risk management. This material is basic to practice and should be covered in the initial orientation. The second section, Liability Issues in Home Care Nursing, provides a more detailed examination of the situations confronting the home care nurse as she practices. This material will be more meaningful to the new nurse after several weeks of home care experience and should be included later in the orientation period. It should also be available for future reference.

Chapter 7 looks at the special considerations of high-tech home care, pediatric home care, and hospice care. These important home care services may not be provided directly by all home health agencies but should be covered as part of initial orientation. All home care nurses will either work with these clients and their families in direct service or in collaboration with other agencies or will need to understand the services to make appropriate referrals.

At the end of the book are several appendices that can be used to clarify material covered in the chapters. Also included is a list of references, as well as a list of additional resources, that can be helpful to the orientation coordinator, new staff nurse, and student nurse.

The Orientation Program

There are many important parts of an orientation program that could not be included in this book. Some are agency-specific (related to personnel forms and procedures), others are ways to measure a nurse's clinical competence. At the beginning of each chapter agency-specific materials that relate to chapter content are listed and should be used if available in the agency. The following list contains additional orientation material that the orientation coordinator/supervisor will want to consider including in the orientation program.

ADDITIONAL AGENCY ORIENTATION MATERIAL CHECKLIST

Personnel
General employee orientation
Review of orientation schedule
Tour of facility/introductions
Work hours and breaks/time off/pay period
Dress code
Mileage procedure

Forms & Procedures
Patient admission and discharge
Verbal orders
Financial/billing forms and information
Updating clinical and personnel information
   Recertification
   Care plan
Medicare denial form
Computer system
   Clinical and/or management systems
Unusual patient situations
   Discharge for safety reasons
   Discharge due to lack of reimbursement source
   Patient refusal of service
   Discharge due to noncompliance with agency policies
Equipment and supplies procedure

Clinical (You may want to develop a skills checklist that can be used as a self-assessment)
Skills and Procedures
   Physical assessment
   Psychosocial assessment
   Medication assessment
   Nutrition assessment
   Practice clinical skills detailed in agency procedure manual

Suggested Format and Content The authors have based the content of this book and the suggested orientation material on the principles of teaching and learning combined with material essential to effective home care nursing practice. The following are items that the authors feel are overriding concerns to be considered when determining how an agency sets up an orientation program for new nursing staff.

1. **An organized orientation program.** Orientation should be structured and organized but not overwhelming. Leave time for questions and discussion as nurses will need time to think about all the information they are receiving. The orientation pace sets the tone for future work in the agency, that is, if it is too slow and unorganized the nurse will believe that is how the entire agency operates. On the other hand, if orientation is rapid and important items that the nurse is later expected to understand are skipped over, distrust evolves and dissatisfaction with the job and agency will soon follow.

2. **Observational visits.** New staff nurses should be sent on a few observational visits beginning **no later than** their third workday. The actual performance of a home visit is a concern to some nurses new to home care, and that concern will block learning until their anxiety is reduced. Once a few home visits are out of the way the nurse is freed up to learn and relate the information to her new position.

3. Getting to know coworkers. Allow time for the nurse to get to know her coworkers throughout the agency, not just in the clinical department. The supervisor might want to arrange for the new nurse to go to lunch with the other nursing staff or host a time (with refreshments) at the end of the workday for the new nurse to meet the entire staff so that she can feel a part of the agency early on.

4. **Timetable.** Most orientation programs are planned over a period of 2 to 4 weeks. The authors suggest that whatever the preference is for length of initial orientation (e.g., 1–4 weeks), there should be time set aside during the probationary period (usually 6 months) to discuss more thoroughly the critical elements of home care nursing, such as agency philosophy, caseload management, productivity, and use of community resources, as well as for the new staff nurse to work with a preceptor. Although these concepts are introduced in the initial orientation, they need to be reinforced and tested throughout the early months of employment.

5. **Orientation to the business office.** The relationship between the nurse and the business office of the home health agency is critical to the success of the agency itself. The nurse's orientation should include scheduled time in the business office, not just a quick walk-through. The authors suggest having the new nurse spend at least a half day working with business office staff at the time of

the month when paperwork is processed for billing. In this way the nurse develops a greater understanding of her role in accurately completing the paperwork involved in home care. The orientation coordinator or personnel department of the agency should also make time in the orientation of business office staff to work with the nurses. A true collegial relationship can be formed, and the operations of the agency will progress more smoothly.

6. **Using a Preceptor.** The use of a preceptor may be useful in socializing a new nurse to the various roles of home care. Many agencies use the term senior nurse to denote those staff who, by virtue of their knowledge, expertise, and seniority have increased responsibilities, some of which are in the orientation area.

A preceptor can be defined as an experienced registered nurse who is selected based on demonstrated proficiency in both clinical and interpersonal skills. She should function as a clinical instructor, professional role model, and resource to the new staff nurse. The preceptor should work with the orientation coordinator and supervisor to assess the learning needs of the new staff nurse, plan and implement an appropriate clinical orientation, and evaluate the clinical performance of the new nurse during the orientation period.

Specific responsibilities should be given to the preceptor and her role in orientation should be acknowledged by title, release from other responsibilities, and financial remuneration. In creating the preceptor role, the criteria outlined in the next column can be useful in choosing staff and in developing evaluation guidelines.

New home care nurses report a positive response to the use of a preceptor who is able to show them the ropes and is readily available to answer questions related to clinical practice as they arise. A new nurse often feels more comfortable coming to her preceptor with minor issues rather than taking the time to ask her supervisor and appearing inadequate to the person who is evaluating her.

Suggested Orientation Schedule The following schedule is a recommended outline of the activities used to orient nurses to home care. This schedule can be used if one or a group of nurses are being oriented to the agency at the same time. The orientation coordinator should set up the schedule keeping in mind the chapters in this book, the agency material listed in the previous section, and the materials suggested at the beginning of each chapter. Each chapter begins with objectives and key concepts that identify the critical

Criteria for Selecting a Preceptor

Professional and Personal Insight
Self confidence
Identifies own strengths and weaknesses and develops ways to address them
Knows when to ask for assistance
Possess constructive empathy
Excellent communication skills
Understands what facilitates communication
A good listener
Ability to identify verbal and nonverbal cues
Approaches people with a non-threatening and non-judgmental attitude
Leadership Abilities
Is enthusiastic
Has a sense of humor
Well organized, yet flexible
Objective and fair
Assertive
Serves as a professional role model
Reality oriented
Respected by peers
Teaching Skills
Knowledgeable of subject to be taught
Ability to use educational resources
Knowledge of adult teaching and learning principles
Possess Expert Theoretical and Clinical Skills
Experience in home care nursing
Is familiar with agency policies and procedures
Able to successfully integrate educational and work values
Has a strong background in nursing theory and its application
Is knowledgeable regarding environmental, cultural, and socioeconomic issues relative to patient care

elements of the orientation program. Whenever an entire chapter or section is assigned, the coordinator should provide an opportunity to discuss the **Test Yourself** questions relating to that material. The orientation coordinator should allocate time each day of the orientation period to meet with the new staff nurse(s) to discuss progress and any questions or problems she(they) may be encountering. Throughout the orientation program, the preceptor has the responsibility of assisting the new staff nurse with visit activities as outlined in agency policy, but the preceptor needs to be careful not to impinge upon supervisory responsibility.

SUGGESTED ORIENTATION SCHEDULE

Week One

- Day 1. (In agency) Chapter 1, process through personnel, Windshield Survey (see Appendix 1)
- Day 2. (In field) New staff nurse accompanies preceptor for entire day, observing all nursing activities
- Day 3. (In agency) Chapter 2, issue bag, read client care record. Schedule appointments with agency personnel (therapy, business office, social work, etc.)
- Day 4. (In field) Joint visits with preceptor. New staff nurse conducts home visit for a client with a care plan established and observes preceptor admit new client to service (Preceptor assists with all documentation, which will be covered Day 5.)
- Day 5. (In agency) Chapter 3, documentation section. Meeting with orientation coordinator to summarize week's activities

Week 2

- Day 1. (In agency) Chapter 4
- Day 2. (In field) Visit clients, at least one of whom has a teaching intervention as part of care plan
- Day 3. (In agency) Chapter 5
- Day 4. (In field) Visit clients
- Day 5. (In field) Visit clients

Week 3

- Day 1. (In field) Visit clients, one admission
- Day 2. (In agency) Chapter 3, quality assurance section and Chapter 6, basic legal considerations section. Meet with quality assurance coodinator
- Day 3. (In field) Visit clients, at least one discharge
- Day 4. (In agency) Work in billing office, Chapter 7, hospice section
- Day 5. (In field) Visit clients

Weeks 4 and 8

If the agency has special programs the nurse will be working with, Chapter 7, which includes high-tech, pediatric home care, and hospice care should be integrated into the orientation program during this part of the orientation. If there are other special programs and community resources with which the nurse will be working, these 5 weeks provide a good opportunity to integrate them into the nurse's workweek. These last 5 weeks are very important in the orientation program and should not be eliminated.

The orientation coordinator should meet with the new staff nurse(s) at least weekly during the fourth through eighth weeks to explore concerns relating to orientation. Time should also be allocated during this period to clarify and reinforce the material covering certain complex areas, such as documentation, quality assurance, contracting, conducting the home visit, use of community resources, and billing procedures. In the seventh or eighth week, the new staff nurse can review material covered in the second section of Chapter 6, legal liability issues. This section examines closely situations confronting the home care nurse that have legal implications and will be more meaningful to the new staff nurse only after several weeks of home care experience.

Organization of the Home Care System

chapter one

OBJECTIVES

Upon completion of this chapter, the reader is prepared to identify:

1. The development and current status of home care in the United States
2. The structure and human resource aspects of home health agencies
3. The external forces that affect the provision of home care
4. Organizations that influence home care services
5. A definition of home care licensure, certification, and accreditation
6. The rights and responsibilities that affect the client and agency relationship

KEY CONCEPTS

- **Definitions of home care**

- **The difference between technical and professional home care**

- **Roles of home care providers**

- **Types of home care reimbursement**

- **Ways to assure quality control**

- **Patient Bill of Rights and Responsibilities**

AGENCY-SPECIFIC MATERIAL NEEDED:

- Mission statement
- Brochure
- Organizational chart
- Orientee's job description
- Patient bill of rights and responsibilities

INTRODUCTION

The 1980s witnessed a rapid increase in the need for home care with the resultant effect being a growth in the number, type, and variety of organizations that provide health services in the home. The dramatic increase in the number of home care providers has been as confusing for health practitioners as it has been for consumers of these services. This chapter will outline the many aspects of the home care field, while the subsequent chapters will look specifically at the field of home care nursing. Definitions of home care and the various external components that affect the field will be discussed. By the end of the chapter, the new home care nurse will better understand the broad field of home care so she can determine where and how her practice fits into this vast field. In no area of nursing practice is the understanding of the larger practice system more important than in that of home care.

DEVELOPMENT OF HOME CARE IN THE UNITED STATES

Home Care—The Past

The root of home care is found in the practice of visiting nursing, which had its beginnings in the United States in the late 1800s. The modern concept of providing nursing care in the home was established by William Rathbone of Liverpool, England, in 1859. Mr. Rathbone, a wealthy businessman and philanthropist, set up a system of visiting nursing after a personal experience when nurses cared for his wife at home before her death. In 1859, with the help of Florence Nightingale, he started a school to train visiting nurses at the Liverpool Infirmary, the graduates of which focused on helping the "sick poor" in their homes (Clemen-Stone, Eigsti, McGuire, 1987).

In the late 1800s the United States experienced rapid growth in its cities, and the waves of immigrants who came to America seeking opportunity played a large role in this change. It is felt that these two social factors were the underlying reasons for the development of visiting nurses in the United States. Like the experiences in England, caring for the ill in their homes focused, from its inception, on the poor. At that time, dismal living and working conditions gave rise to problems with hygiene and increases in various illnesses.

Visiting nurse associations (VNAs) in the United States, like their English counterparts, were established by groups of people who wanted to assist the poor to improve their health. Buffalo, NY, Boston, and Philadelphia developed visiting nurse services during 1885 and 1886 and focused on caring for the middle-class sick as well as the poor (Clemen-Stone et al., 1987).

During World War II, as physicians made fewer home visits and focused instead on their offices and hospitals, the home care movement grew, with nurses providing most of the health and illness care in the home. In 1946, Montefiore Hospital in New York City developed a posthospital acute care program, and convalescent home care was started (Mundinger, 1983).

From these early beginnings through the mid-1960s, VNAs were developed in major cities, small towns, and counties throughout the country. During that period much of their work focused on providing health and illness services to the poor in their homes with most of the acute care given to patients in a hospital setting. With the passage of Medicare legislation through the Social Security Act in 1965, home care, almost solely provided by VNAs, became more frequently used since it was a benefit provided to elderly patients who participated in the Medicare program.

Home Care—The Present

In the early 1980s, to curb the increasing hospital costs incurred by the Medicare program and the increasing numbers of elderly patients needing hospitalization, diagnostic-related groupings (DRGs) were phased in over a 4-year period in hospitals nationwide. Two results of the implementation of the DRG system were a decrease in a patient's length of stay in the hospital and an increase in the use of home care services to these patients. Also, since Medicare would not cover hospitalization for some conditions, many patients were not admitted to a hospital, and the needed care was, therefore, provided in the home by a home care agency. Following the federal government's lead with the Medicare program, Medicaid programs, which are administered individually by the states, private insurance companies, and other payors who cover home health services, also began restricting payments for hospitalizations, thus increasing the need for home care services.

Home care, home health care, and home health agency can be confusing terms, even to the providers of the care. Home care and home health care have been used synonymously by those working in the field and will be used the same way in this book. So, how exactly is home care defined today?

Contemporary Definitions of Home Care

The following list represents definitions of home care developed by leading professional and trade associations in the field.

- Medicare Definition. Illness care
- National Association for Home Care (NAHC) Definition.

"Services to the recovering, disabled or chronically ill person providing for treatment and/or effective functioning in the home environment. Home care can also assist in the provision of services to adults and children in danger of abuse or neglect. Generally, home care is appropriate whenever a person needs assistance that cannot be easily or effectively provided only by family members or friends on an ongoing basis for a short or long period of time" (National Association for Home Care, 1987).

- American Hospital Association Definition (Friedman, 1986). Home care constitutes:

Medical care and supervision	Speech therapy
Nursing care and supervision	Inhalation therapy
Social work services	Medical technician services
Physical therapy	Appliance, equipment, and sterile supply services
Occupational therapy	Pharmaceutical services
Nutritional guidance	Transportation for patient and equipment
Laboratory and radiology services	Homemaker and home health aide services

- American Medical Association Definition.

"The provision of nursing care, social work, therapies, vocational and social services, and homemaker-health aide services may be included as basic components of home health care. The provision of these needed services to the patient at home constitutes a logical extension of the physician's therapeutic responsibility. At the physician's request and under his medical direction, personnel who provide these home health care services operate as a team in assessing and developing the home health care plan" (Health and Public Policy Committee, 1986).

- Consumer's Union Definition.

"People care at home. It is diagnosis, treatment, monitoring, rehabilitation, and supportive care provided at home, rather than in an impersonal hospital, nursing home, or other institution. At best, home care is holistic, providing in-home health, social, and other human services that can help you as a whole person, not just as a 'patient' " (Nassif, 1985).

Although the home care definitions presented thus far may tend to confuse the reader, they do represent the divergent opinions of home care and leave room for further discussion and clarification. This broad notion of exactly what home care involves indicates that home care is evolving and that providers, payors, and clients have far to go in clarifying the role and function of home care and home care providers.

For the purpose of this book, home care will be used as the term that describes the broad spectrum of professional and technical services delivered in the home. The authors do believe, however, that there is a distinct difference between the professional and technical home care services that are provided to clients.

The Difference Between Professional and Technical Home Care

Professional Home Care is practice-driven, that is, the boundaries of practice are determined by professional standards with a basis in scientific theory and research. The foundation for this type of practice is strong and is provided by professionals with licenses, certifications, or specific qualifications. Nursing, therapy, social work, and paraprofessional services, such as home health aides, are examples of professional home care practice.

Technical Home Care is product-driven, often with a zeal for bottom line profits, and does not always consider what is the best for the client. The providers of this care do not have standards or regulations that govern how they provide home care. Only reimbursement guidelines, which simply outline what will and won't be covered by third party payors, exist. Durable medical equipment (DME) suppliers, oxygen providers, and other equipment home delivery providers make up this category (Humphrey, 1988)

This book focuses on the **professional** practice of home care and home care nursing, so the technical aspects of home care are discussed only briefly. Professional services, which are primarily for the acutely ill and that are skilled, short-term, and intermittent is the emphasis of this book. In the delivery of a professional model of home care, nursing is the foundation of the entire system and will be discussed in following chapters. It is up to the home care nurse to examine her role continually and determine how she is to practice this specialized field of nursing in the larger home care and health care system.

THE HOME HEALTH AGENCY

The Medicare Conditions of Participation for Home Health Agencies define a home health agency as "a public agency or a private organization . . . primarily engaged in providing skilled nursing services and other therapeutic services" (Harris, 1988). The following list will describe briefly the many types of agencies that provide home health care.

Types of Agencies

Voluntary Agencies. Home health agencies (HHAs) that do not depend on state and local tax revenues but are financed primarily with nontax funds, such as donations, endowments, United Way contributions, and third-party insurance provider payments (Medicare, Medicaid, private insurance), are referred to as voluntary agencies. An example is the visiting nurse associations.

Voluntary agencies are usually governed by a voluntary board of directors and are considered to be community based since they provide services within a well-defined geographic location or community. Whereas in the past, voluntary agencies were assured of receiving almost all the home care referrals in their community, the proliferation of other agencies has eroded their traditional referral base and put them in a competitive mode with other home care providers.

Private, Proprietary Agencies. Private home health agencies can be for-profit and not-for-profit organizations. Most private home health agencies are for-profit, known as proprietary agencies. Private agencies can be governed by individual owner(s), but many of the large for-profit home health agencies are part of national chains that are administered through corporate headquarters.

Proprietary agencies plan to make a profit on the home care services they provide, either for the private individuals who own them or for their stockholders. Some proprietary agencies participate in the Medicare program, and some do not. While revenues are generated by some proprietary agencies through third-party payors, such as Medicare and private insurance, others rely on "private-pay" (clients who pay their own money). Many agencies also provide hospital staffing services in addition to home care.

Institution-Based Agencies. A health care organization, such as a hospital, may operate a separate department as a home health agency. This agency would then be governed by the sponsoring organization's board of directors or trustees. The referrals to this agency usually come from the sponsoring institution, and the missions of the home health agency and the "parent" institution are similar.

Governmental Agencies. Governmental home health agencies are called official agencies and are created and given their power through statutes enacted by legislation. Home health services are frequently provided by the nursing divisions of state or local health departments and may or may not combine the home care services (care of the sick) with their traditional public health nursing (preventive) services.

Traditional public health nursing services provided through an official agency are communicable disease investigation, health promotion, disease prevention, and environmental health services, as well as maternal–child health and family planning. Fiscal and administrative support for these agencies is the responsibility of the city, county, or state government or a combination of the three.

Homemaker–Home Health Aide Agencies. Agencies that provide homemaker–home health aide services exclusively are usually private and derive their reimbursement from direct payment by the client or private insurance policies. They may also be governed by individual owners or corporate headquarters.

Hospice. The National Hospice Organization (1984) defines a hospice as an agency in which "services are provided by a medically supervised interdisciplinary team of professionals and volunteers for terminally ill clients." A more in-depth discussion of hospice care is found in Chapter 7.

Other Home Care Providers. As is evident from the broad scope of home care definitions mentioned earlier, other types of home care services can be provided by companies that perform a technical, house call function rather than a professional home care one. Usually these companies provide durable medical equipment (DME), high-technology services (e.g., ventilators, total parenteral nutrition), and other services to assist clients in their home. These home care providers do not deliver any professional services in the home, such as nursing, therapy, or social work, or paraprofessional assistance, such as homemakers and home health aides.

PERSONNEL IN A HOME HEALTH AGENCY

The organizational structure of a home health agency varies by type, size, geographical location and levels of accountability. The following discussion will describe briefly the positions, functions, and roles of the typical positions found in the three areas of a home health agency: administration, management, and staff.

Administration

The following three positions make up the basic administrative personnel of a home health agency. Various titles can be given to the positions, but the responsibilities remain the same. If the agency is very large there may be more top administrators with various roles identified.

Executive Director or Chief Executive Officer (CEO). The CEO is responsible for the total administration of the agency and reports to the board of directors, owner, or corporate headquarters.

Assistant Director or Chief Operating Officer (COO). The COO is responsible for the day-to-day operations of the agency and is usually someone with a professional clinical background in one of the services provided by the agency. Most often that background is nursing, since most of the service provided is nursing. The COO reports to the CEO.

Finance Director or Chief Financial Officer (CFO). The CFO is responsible for the total financial operations of the agency. This administrator usually supervises the business office and reports to the CEO.

Management

The various management roles in a home health agency are the ones most determined by size, type, and programs delivered by the agency. If programs or services are offered beyond the basic ones found in most home health agencies (e.g., nursing; physical, speech, and occupational therapy; social work; home health aide), there will be a management person assigned to each program. The following is a list of typical management positions related to the clinical functions of a home health agency. The business office role and functions will be covered at the end of this section.

Director of Clinical Services. The professional in this top management position, which oversees the personnel delivering the various program services of the agency, is really the supervisor's supervisor and may have several program directors and clinical supervisors reporting to him or her. The responsibility for maintaining the agency's professional standards of patient care and compliance with various regulatory guidelines lies with this position. This director is comparable to the hospital director of nursing who reviews every aspect of the agency operations that affect patient care. In smaller agencies this function may be assumed by the clinical nursing supervisor(s).

Nursing Supervisor or Clinical Coordinator. This supervisor is comparable to the head nurse in a hospital who usually assigns and schedules professional personnel, and oversees and helps coordinate the care given by the nursing staff. The supervisor monitors the care given by all staff members working in the patient's care plan and is the link between staff and higher level management and administration.

Intake Coordinator or Home Care Coordinator. The manager at this level processes the initial requests to the agency for home care and may be a nurse or social worker, with nonprofessional clerical workers as assistants.

Home Health Aide Supervisor. Most agencies employ someone in this management position that oversees the personnel functions of the home health aides. Instruction and supervision of a home health aide on direct client care in the home is provided by the nurse assigned to the clients. Further discussion of this is found in Chapter Five. The home health aide supervisor works with the nurses to coordinate and evaluate client care provided by the paraprofessionals and also directs the in-service, scheduling, and personnel-related issues of the home health aides.

Special Supervisors. As mentioned earlier, there may be supervisors of special programs and services provided by a home health agency. Typically, a person must supervise the services delivered by the therapy and social work departments. If the agency provides special programs to patient groups such as maternal–child health services, AIDS, and mental health, one supervisor may be assigned to oversee all those programs.

Staff

Since the staff of a home health agency is mostly determined by the type of services provided, the following list will cover staff found in a typical home health agency, regardless of type.

Nurses. Just like nursing roles that are delivered in most health care settings, home care has several types of positions that deliver nursing care.

Registered Nurse. These nurses may be associate degree, diploma-, or BSN-prepared professionals with responsibilities often tied to their level of education. Most home care agencies feel that a BSN is best prepared to deliver the broad scope of skilled nursing services to their clients. These nurses function in the mode of delivery determined by the agency, that is, primary care, team, or case management. Many RNs now have specialized skills that enable them to work with high-tech clients or clients who need long-term rehabilitation in the home.

Nurse Practitioner. This nurse may provide total client care, supervise others in difficult cases related to their specialty, or direct a special program. For example, a pediatric nurse practitioner may not only deliver direct care to the agency's pediatric patients but may act as a consultant to staff RNs to develop a care plan for their pediatric clients.

Enterostomal Therapist (ET). An agency may have an ET on staff who will provide direct care to clients or act as a consultant to staff members whose clients have bowel or bladder problems or wound management problems.

Licensed Practical Nurse (LPN)—Called Licensed Vocational Nurse (LVN) in California and Texas. The specific skills that an LPN can deliver to a home care client and the type of reimbursement are governed by the state nurse practice acts, state licensure laws for home health agencies, and the policies of various reimbursement sources.

Therapists

Physical Therapist (PT). The PT delivers skilled care that involves assessment for assistive devices, relative to rehabilitation and safety, that can be used in the home, performs therapy procedures for the client, and teaches the client or family to assist in treatment. The PT usually works with a client who has limited mobility and is unable to go out of the home for therapy. The client's diagnosis must reflect the need for PT services.

Occupational Therapist (OT). This therapist provides care that is concerned with peak function, focusing on improving physical, mental, or social abilities. It is often difficult to decide when a client needs physical or occupational therapy, and the assessment should be made by the therapy department in collaboration with a nursing supervisor and the physician.

Speech Therapist (ST). The ST provides speech therapy for clients whose diagnosis or condition indicates a need for such therapy.

Respiratory Therapist (RT). Some home health agencies work on a contractual basis with respiratory therapists for clients who have a diagnosis related to their respiratory function. This relationship is especially important with clients who are on ventilator support, and often the RT works with the DME in providing not only the technical products and services (e.g., ventilator, oxygen) but also the professional treatment as well.

Other Clinical Staff

Social Worker (SW). Traditionally, social workers help clients and their families identify needs and make referrals to community resources that can be helpful. In home care the social work function also includes assisting with applications for services and providing financial assistance information.

Dietitians. These staff members provide diet and nutrition counseling to clients with special needs. If an agency has this service available it is usually on a contractual basis, since the direct service of a dietitian is not a reimbursable home care service.

Paraprofessionals. A home health agency usually provides the service of home health aides and, depending on the type of agency, homemaker services. Although these positions are separate, their functions overlap in many areas. The rule of thumb is that a home health aide may perform some of the duties of a homemaker (related to household tasks) but a homemaker is not qualified to provide the hands-on care of a home health aide.

Home Health Aide (HHA). At most agencies a home health aide performs three general services: (1) personal care, (2) basic nursing tasks (as opposed to skilled), and (3) incidental homemaking. The home health agency will have a list of the "basic" nursing procedures a home health aide may perform, and you will need to become familiar with these so you can supervise the aides appropriately. Basic nursing tasks include taking vital signs, selected treatments, and assisting the patient with self-administered medications. State laws prohibit aides from administering medications.

Homemaker (HM). The bulk of the work a homemaker provides is light housekeeping, such as washing the dishes, doing the laundry, preparing light meals and changing the linens. Homemakers may also do shopping and pick up medications for the client. Homemakers never perform heavy housework and only under very strict guidance may assist the client directly with a minor aspect of personal care.

Business Office Staff. The business office of a home health agency is an integral part of the organization's ability to deliver services to clients. A home health agency cannot perform efficiently and effectively without a sound business department that works well with clinical staff. Never in your nursing career are you called upon to become involved with the financial aspects of your clients' care as you will be in home care. Throughout your orientation you will learn how to relate to the business department of your agency and what systems are in place for the processing of visit and financial information. As you look at the organizational structure, position titles, roles, and responsibilities of all departments in your agency, be sure to be clear also on the functions and personnel who work in the business office; they will help you get your job done more efficiently.

ENVIRONMENTAL INFLUENCES ON HOME CARE

Many factors outside of organizational structure and the professional responsibilities of providers influence the way home care is provided. Since the beginning of home care was based on societal trends, it is important to look at the current social environments to understand better how and why home care is practiced today.

Environmental Aspects

Home care nursing is practiced within the context of the larger health care system. The nature of home care, providing care to individuals and families in their homes, indicates that there are many aspects in the external environment that affect the way nurses are able to deliver care. The following list outlines the main external factors a nurse must be aware of to work in the field of home care.

Reimbursement

Federal Government. Medicare (Title 18 of the Social Security Act) represents an effort by the federal government to provide national health insurance to an across-the-board population based on chronological age and some other considerations. It is an **insurance program** that almost everyone over 65 years of age is eligible for, regardless of income. It also includes persons under 65 years of age who are disabled and are receiving Social Security benefits.

Medicare accounts for more than 60% of all payments for home delivered services. The system is set up to operate uniformly throughout all 50 states, the American commonwealth (Puerto Rico), and American protectorates (Virgin Islands of the United States). The Medicare program is administered by the Health Care Financing Administration (HCFA), a branch of the Department of Health and Human Services (HHS). The Health Care Financing Administration (HCFA) is responsible for overseeing the entire Medicare program, which governs how and what services are reimbursed by Medicare. The Medicare home health benefit is regulated by HCFA. The home health regulations set forth by HCFA have a great impact on how the home care nurse practices if she is caring for a Medicare client. The policies and regulations set by HCFA in the clinical and reimbursement areas are often followed by other payors, such as Medicaid and private insurance (Harris, 1988).

Although the administration of Medicare is controlled by HCFA, payments to agencies on behalf of the program are handled by a *fiscal intermediary* (FI). The FI is usually an insurance company that has a contract with HCFA to see that the regulations are carried out appropriately by providers (home health agencies), and to issue payments on behalf of the Medicare beneficiary (the patient). The documentation section in this book (Chapter 3) outlines Medicare requirements for home care, documentation necessary to indicate that care is covered, and how services are paid by the FI.

State Government. Medicaid (Title 19 of the Social Security Act), a *public assistance program*, is a federally assisted state program that provides health care benefits to needy and low-income persons. Medicaid eligibility and coverage criteria vary from state to state, and you should review the Medicaid home care regulations for your state with your supervisor. The Medicaid program accounts for more than 20% of all home health agency funding nationwide.

Commercial Insurance. Companies, such as Blue Cross, AEtna, Prudential, and the Travelers, provide varying degrees of home care coverage for the people they insure. The health insurance industry is rapidly recognizing the savings that can be realized by the use of home care services instead of institutional care, but getting coverage for clients who have private insurance is often as difficult as it can be for other types of payments, such as Medicare. Since commercial insurance coverage varies so much from client to client, it is best that someone in the agency determine exactly what home care coverage the client has upon admission to the home health agency. Check with your supervisor on the agency's policy for dealing with private insurance clients.

Indigent Care. Delivering home care to clients who have no payment source has long been the mission of the nonprofit home health agencies, such as visiting nurse associations. Often called free care, it is important that you, as a home care nurse, understand that the care is not free—someone is paying for it, just not the client. If an agency lets the amount of free care exceed the financial resources available for providing subsidized care, the agency can face a potentially catastrophic financial loss, which could jeopardize the future of the agency. Check your agency's policy on free and reduced fee care.

Other Reimbursement Programs and Payment Sources. There are many other programs existing nationally and on state or local levels that have been designed to assist home care clients who fall between the cracks of the Medicare and Medicaid programs. These programs, however, account for only 5% to 10% of the total monies spent nationwide for home care.

Private cash payors make up another payment source to the home health agency, but only to a very limited degree for the traditional services provided (nursing; physical, speech, and occupational therapy; social work; and home health aide). Private pay clients usually pay for the services of a private duty RN, or for a home health aide beyond what is covered by another payor. They also pay for other services desired by the client that go beyond what is covered by a third party payor. Rarely do clients pay directly for the minimum traditional services provided when they are acutely ill.

Home Care Organizations

The following is a list of the organizations that represent home care providers along with a brief description of their purposes.

National Association for Home Care. The National Association for Home Care (NAHC) is the major organization that represents the broad spectrum of home health services on a national level. Formed in 1982 by a merger of National Association of Home Health Agencies (NAHHA) and the Council of Home Health Agencies/Community Health Services (CHHA/CHS), NAHC is governed by a board of directors and has four types of membership: provider, associate, allied, and individual.

Provider membership is open to home health agencies, homemaker–home health aide organizations, and hospices. Associate membership is for those who work in the home care industry but are not direct providers (e.g., law, accounting, and consulting firms). Allied membership is for related health groups with an interest in the field of home care, such as schools of nursing, while individual membership is for individual professionals working for a provider member who wish to join on their own. The purposes of NAHC are

1. To represent the interests of those Americans described as being on the "fringes of life"—the elderly, millions of fragile children facing major health problems, and the disabled
2. To heighten the political visibility of home care services
3. To affect legislative and regulatory processes impinging on home care services
4. To gather and disseminate data on the home care industry
5. To promote home care as a viable component of the health care delivery system
6. To foster, develop, and promote high standards of client care in home care services
7. To provide an organized and unified voice of home care provider organizations
8. To disseminate information and provide for the exchange of information with those interested in home care services and total health care
9. To interpret home care services for governmental and private sector bodies that affect the delivery and financing of home care services
10. To collaborate with state organizations representing home care interests and other organizations at the local, state, and national levels
11. To initiate, sponsor, and promote educational programs for and with providers and consumers of home care
12. To initiate, sponsor, and promote research related to home care services, directly or indirectly, through grants, contracts, or other arrangements
13. To engage in any and all other activities permitted by law for the promotion of the association's purposes, and
14. To foster a mutually beneficial relationship with other organizations interested in the well-being of the home care population.

The National Association for Home Care has several associated organizations, which will be briefly listed here.

Foundation for Hospice and Homecare. This is a nonprofit charitable organization the goals of which are to promote high standards, promote research, and educate the public concerning matters of health and social policy related to hospice and home care issues.

National HomeCaring Council Division. This national standard-setting body for the homemaker–home health aide field is a division of the Foundation for Hospice and Homecare. It also has a nationally recognized accreditation program for homemaker–home health aide programs.

Hospice Association of America. This association was formed to focus greater attention nationally on hospice issues.

National Association for Physicians in Home Care (NAPHC). The National Association for Home Care established the NAPHC to provide a forum for physicians who participate in home care services.

State Home Care Associations. Many states have home care associations that exist for varied purposes. The activities of a state association include involvement in educational activities, government relations, programs that focus on state legislative and regulatory activities related to home care, communication to members in the form of newsletters and bulletins, and development of any other services to meet the needs of its membership.

VNA of America. Another organization that represents a sector of home care providers, the visiting nurse associations, is the Visiting Nurse Associations of America (VNAA). The purposes of this organization are fostering communication and cooperation among individual VNAs, promoting a national image, and pooling resources for marketing, advertising, and other operational needs.

Certification, Licensing, and Accreditation

Medicare Conditions of Participation. The regulations that govern how a home health agency must be administered to participate in the Medicare program are called Conditions of Participation. As a staff nurse your main responsibility is to know these conditions exist and to understand that policies, procedures, and billing practices are often dictated by these regulations. Although the responsibility for adherence to the conditions is ultimately up to the managers and administrators of your agency, it is up to everyone on staff, especially the home care nurse, to see that policies are followed.

State Licensing Laws. Most states have licensure laws for home health agencies that set specific requirements about staffing, policies and practices, and set minimal operating standards for various services and programs. The licensure requirements are closely linked to Medicare's Conditions of Participation and usually there is a connection between a state licensing and the agency being a Medicare certified agency. For example, state licensing requirements may be seen as exceeding the minimum set for Medicare certification, and an agency could become both certified for Medicare and state licensed at the same time.

If a home health agency meets certain conditions put forth in the licensure law, it will receive a license; if not, the agency will not be permitted to operate until the standards in the law are met. As a licensed agency, an on-site licensure visit takes place at certain intervals. You will likely be involved in some aspect of the licensure visit under the direction of your supervisor. Check with your supervisor for the local licensure law provisions that affect you.

Accreditation. There are two organizations that accredit home health agencies throughout the country, the Community Health Accreditation Program (CHAP), through the National League for Nursing (NLN), and the Home Care Accreditation Program, through the Joint Commission of Accreditation of Healthcare Organizations (JCAHO). Both programs are voluntary and are used by agencies to further define the issue of quality home care to their community and clients. Some reimbursement sources (insurance companies, HMOs, etc.) and consumer groups (e.g., American Association of Retired Persons) may recognize participation in JCAHO or CHAP as a requirement for their programs, thus making accreditation essential for agencies who want to serve clients from these groups.

The CHAP program through the NLN broadens the accreditation process that the League has implemented over the past 25 years for community health nursing agencies. The program objectives look at quality issues and identify standards that are used by the organization to go beyond the minimum criteria for patient safety set by many organizations.

The Joint Commission on Accreditation of Healthcare Organizations (JCAHO) is a private, not-for-profit organization dedicated to promoting quality health care through a voluntary accreditation process. Formerly focusing on accreditation of inpatient facilities, the commission recently broadened its scope to include home health agencies by developing home care and hospice standards. The accreditation process of the commission is based on these standards and involves submission of an application form to the commission with agency material followed by an on-site survey of the organization conducted by surveyors employed by the commission. Following the review, the agency is notified of its accreditation status. The process is similar for hospice organizations, many of which may be affiliate agencies of the home health agency being reviewed.

Ethical Standards

Home Care Patient Bill of Rights and Responsibilities. The National Association for Home Care has established a national code of ethics for its membership with the goal of informing the general public as to what ethical conduct for home health agencies and their employees involves. Recent federal legislation mandates that home health agencies participating in the Medicare program have a "patient bill of rights

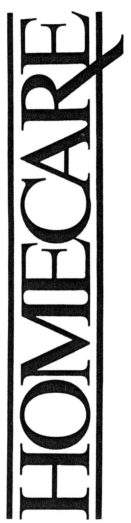

HOMECARE

BILL OF RIGHTS*

Home care consumers (clients) have a right to be notified in writing of their rights and obligations before treatment is begun. The client's family or guardian may exercise the client's rights when the client has been judged incompetent. Home care providers have an obligation to protect and promote the rights of their clients, including the following rights.

Clients and Providers Have a Right to Dignity and Respect

Home care clients and their formal caregivers have a right to mutual respect and dignity. Caregivers are prohibited from accepting personal gifts and borrowing from clients.

Clients have the right:
- to have relationships with home care providers that are based on honesty and ethical standards of conduct;
- to be informed of the procedure they can follow to lodge complaints with the home care provider about the care that is, or fails to be, furnished, and regarding a lack of respect from property (to lodge complaints with us call _____);
- to know about the disposition of such complaints;
- to voice their grievances without fear of discrimination or reprisal for having done this; and
- to be advised of the telephone number and hours of operation of the state's home health comment line. The hours are _____ and the number is _____.

Decisionmaking

Clients have the right:
- to be notified in writing of the care that is to be furnished, the types (disciplines) of the caregivers who will furnish the care and the frequency of the visits that are proposed to be furnished;
- to be advised of any change in the plan of care before the change is made;
- to participate in the planning of the care and in planning changes in the care, and to be advised that they have the right to do so; and
- to refuse services or request a change in caregiver without fear of reprisal or discrimination.

The home care provider or the client's physician may be forced to refer the client to another source of care if the client's refusal to comply with the plan of care threatens to compromise the provider's commitment to quality care.

Privacy

Clients have the right:

- to confidentiality with regard to information about their health, social and financial circumstances and about what takes place in the home; and
- to expect the home care provider to release information only as required by law or authorized by the client.

Financial Information

Clients have the right:

- to be informed of the extent to which payment may be expected from Medicare, Medicaid or any other payor known to the home care provider;
- to be informed of the charges that will not be covered by Medicare;
- to be informed of the charges for which the client may be liable;
- to receive this information, orally and in writing, within fifteen working days of the date the home care provider becomes aware of any changes in charges; and
- to have access, upon request, to all bills for service the client has received regardless of whether they are paid out-of-pocket or by another party.

Quality of Care

Clients have the right:

- to receive care of the highest quality;
- in general, to be admitted by a home care provider only if it has the resources needed to provide the care safely, and at the required level of intensity, as determined by a professional assessment; however, a provider with less than optimal resources may nevertheless admit the client if a more appropriate provider is not available, but only after fully informing the client of its limitations and the lack of suitable alternative arrangements; and
- to be told what to do in the case of an emergency.

Quality of Care

The home care provider shall assure that:

- all medically related home care is provided in accordance with the physicians' orders and that a plan of care specifies the services to be provided and their frequency and duration; and
- all medically related personal care is provided by an appropriately trained homemaker-home health aide who is supervised by a nurse or other qualified home care professional.

*In 1982, the National Association for Home Care adopted a comprehensive Code of Ethics to which all members subscribed. Among the elements in this Code was a clients' Bill of Rights similar to the rights outlined in this document. In 1987, Congress enacted a provision requiring home care agencies to inform clients of these rights.
From the National Association for Home Care, 1990, with permission.

Figure 1–1 Home Care Bill of Rights

and responsibilities." National trends indicate that the federal government will soon mandate specific ethical standards that will guarantee consumers certain rights while protecting the quality of home care they receive.

The NAHC Bill of Rights (Fig. 1–1) is helpful in understanding the rights of clients and families to quality home care. A home health agency may add any other rights they feel are applicable to their clients and may add responsibilities that the client and family must assume to receive home care. Listing both client rights and responsibilities emphasizes the active role clients and families must play in home

care. An example of a client's responsibility might be the requirement to have supportive coverage when agency personnel are not present.

It is important that the new home care nurse understand generally the many aspects involved in the home care system. This chapter has outlined the major aspects common to all home care agencies (e.g., types of agencies, personnel, and environmental influences that affect practice). This information sets the stage for the rest of the book, which examines in detail the role and function of the home care nurse as she works in the larger home health system.

TEST YOURSELF

1. State five aspects of the development of home care in the United States discussed in this chapter that you found interesting.

2. Based on your reading, develop your definition of home care.

3. In what type of home health agency do you work?

4. How does your job fit into the mission of the agency?

5. Name two types of home care reimbursement mechanisms and the populations they serve.

6. Does your agency belong to the NAHC? If yes, what are the benefits you/they derive?

7. Is your agency licensed? Certified? Accredited? If yes, by whom?

8. Discuss the similarities and differences between the NAHC Bill of Rights and Responsibilities and your agency's.

The Specialty of Home Care Nursing

OBJECTIVES

Upon completion of this chapter the reader is prepared to identify:

1. The definition of home care nursing
2. The purpose of home care standards
3. The roles and functions of the home care nurse
4. How the nursing process is implemented in home care nursing practice
5. Universal blood and body fluid precautions as described by the CDC
6. Measures used to control communicable diseases in the home
7. Steps in a home visit
8. Criteria used to determine a patient's discharge from home care

KEY CONCEPTS

- **The definition of home care nursing**

- **The home care nurse as coordinator of services**

- **The effect of reimbursement on home care nursing practice**

- **Setting patient-centered goals and priorities**

- **The use of universal precautions in home care**

- **How to do a home visit**

AGENCY-SPECIFIC MATERIAL NEEDED:

- New staff nurse's job description
- Intra- and interagency referral form
- Listing of community resources with phone numbers
- Local telephone book, including Yellow Pages
- Blank patient care record, including intake form
- Other related information regarding clinical record system (e.g., manual)

- Standardized care plans (if used)
- Map of service area
- Safety policies
- Agency procedure regarding Universal Precautions
- Nursing bag and contents
- Criteria for discharge and discharge summary procedure

INTRODUCTION

Chapter One outlines the many aspects of home care as a broad field that provides both technical and professional services to people in their homes. This chapter serves as an introduction to the focus of this book, that is the provision of **professional** home care nursing services. Home care nursing is a specialized practice area within nursing, and this chapter will outline the numerous components of the role and function of a home care nurse, the nursing process applied to home care, and how to do a home visit.

Before exploring the many aspects of the home care nursing role, it is important to answer the question, What is home care nursing?

HOME CARE NURSING—WHAT IS IT?

Home care nursing is a unique field of nursing practice that focuses on caring for the sick in the home. This unique field of practice requires a synthesis of community health nursing principles with the theory and practice of medical/surgical, maternal–child, and mental health nursing. Home care nursing is provided to clients experiencing an illness outside the confines of an acute care hospital. Home care nurses care for acute and chronic clients of all ages, those who have procedures and treatments conducted in their home, and those who wish to live out the final stages of life in their home rather than in an institution.

Home care nursing, especially since the inception of Medicare, has become known as the provision of care to ill persons in the home as evidenced by the definitions outlined in Chapter 1. Many agencies call their home care program, Care of the Ill (COI), to denote this specific kind of patient as compared with those clients who are primarily receiving health promotion/illness prevention interventions. Clearly, home care nursing is much more than just the provision of medical/surgical nursing in the home.

The client cared for by the home care nurse is the individual patient, their family, and significant others. Caring for an ill individual at home is complex and requires that the nurse consider numerous factors related to the patient's family, home and community. Also to care for a home care client professionally the nurse must understand how the environmental, psychosocial, economic, cultural, and personal health-related factors affect the client's illness and their ability to meet the goals outlined in the plan of care. This broad approach of caring for individuals,

families, and communities is the cornerstone of community health nursing practice.

Community health nurses are experts on intervening with families and communities to maximize the effect of the medical and nursing regimen on the client's care. To deliver home care services effectively, the nurse must be familiar with principles of community health nursing and with the principles underlying medical/surgical, maternal–child, and mental health nursing practice. These practice areas are used together by the home care nurse to provide comprehensive quality nursing services to clients in their home.

In the current regulatory and economic climate in health care, it is increasingly difficult for the home care nurse to practice the community health nursing role with clients. Reimbursement sources focus on medical diagnoses and often are not supportive of what they perceive is the "extra" care (beyond basic medical/surgical care) a client may need. For example, a client who needs a dressing change may also be having difficulty coping with her diagnosis and prognosis and should be able to discuss it with the nurse with the possibility of being referred to other agencies for the necessary counseling. The extra time needed to integrate this supportive care is difficult to deliver when the nurse is asked to justify reimbursement for service by focusing on the direct care given to the wound. Intervention in areas other than wound care are not supported by reimbursement sources and often not by others in the home care area.

It is important that, in this environment, the home care nurse continue to provide a comprehensive approach to client care (relating to all areas of nursing practice) and act as a client advocate in justifying this care as essential, not extra. The focus of nursing care is the treatment of human responses. Home care nursing demands that the varied human responses seen in home care clients are addressed in a holistic framework so the client and family can be assisted to thoroughly reach their goals.

Definition of Home Care Nursing

Although many sources discuss the aspects of home care nursing, there is no consensus on a definition. For the purpose of this book, the following definition will be used:

Home care nursing is the provision of nursing care to acute and chronically ill clients of all ages in their home while integrating community health nursing principles that focus on the environmental, psychosocial, economic, cultural, and personal health factors affecting an individual's and family's health status.

HOME CARE NURSING STANDARDS

An essential aspect of home care nursing that sets it apart from the services of *technical* home care providers is that of a practice based on professional standards. The American Nurses' Association has produced Home Care Nursing Standards to fulfill the profession's obligation to provide a means of improving the quality of care provided to consumers. Standards reflect the current state of knowledge in the field and are the basis for characterizing, measuring, and providing guidance in achieving quality care. The home care standards are based on the ANA Standards of Community Health Nursing and are to be used with that document to base nursing service practice in home health agencies. The standards, without their interpretive statements, are found in Figure 2–1.

The standards reflect two levels of practice: that of the generalist prepared at the baccalaureate level and that of the specialist prepared at the graduate level. These standards outline levels of professional nursing practice to be achieved by the nurse and should be reviewed with your supervisor early in your orientation. As the home care nurse goes through the orientation, she should look for the ways her agency integrates the standards in the many areas of practice and the agency's policies.

Standard I. Organization of Home Health Services
All home health services are planned, organized, and directed by a master's-prepared professional nurse with experience in community health and administration.

Standard II. Theory
The nurse applies theoretical concepts as a basis for decisions in practice.

Standard III. Data Collection
The nurse continuously collects and records data that are comprehensive, accurate, and systematic.

Standard IV. Diagnosis
The nurse uses health assessment data to determine nursing diagnoses.

Standard V. Planning
The nurse develops care plans that establish goals. The care plan is based on nursing diagnoses and incorporates therapeutic, preventive, and rehabilitative nursing actions.

Standard VI. Intervention
The nurse, guided by the care plan, intervenes to provide comfort, to restore, improve, and promote health, to prevent complications and sequelae of illness, and to effect rehabilitation.

Standard VII. Evaluation
The nurse continually evaluates the client's and family's responses to interventions in order to determine progress toward goal attainment and to revise the data base, nursing diagnosis, and plan of care.

Standard VIII. Continuity of Care
The nurse is responsible for the client's appropriate and uninterrupted care along the health care continuum, and therefore, uses discharge planning, case management, and coordination of community resources.

Standard IX. Interdisciplinary Collaboration
The nurse initiates and maintains a liaison relationship with all appropriate health care providers to assure that all efforts effectively complement one another.

Standard X. Professional Development
The nurse assumes responsibility for professional development and contributes to the professional growth of others.

Standard XI. Research
The nurse participates in research activities that contribute to the profession's continuing development of knowledge of home health care.

Standard XII. Ethics
The nurse uses the code for nurses established by the American Nurses' Association as a guide for ethical decision making in practice.

Reprinted with permission from Standards of Home Health Nursing Practice, *1986, American Nurses' Association, Kansas City, Mo.*

Figure 2–1. The American Nurses' Association Home Care Nursing Standards.

ROLE AND FUNCTION OF THE HOME CARE NURSE

Although there is a great deal of similarity between the nursing practice of home care nurses and their colleagues who work in a hospital, there are many roles and functions a home care nurse must assume that are different from the nursing roles assumed in an institutional setting. This section will examine the roles and functions of the home care nurse, focusing on the **differences** between home care practice and institutional practice.

Providing Direct Care

Direct care is defined as the actual nursing interventions delivered in the home visit. Direct care activities include **assessment, performing a procedure, and teaching.** Assessing a client's cardiovascular status, changing a dressing, or teaching the client and family about a new diet or medication would be examples of the three direct care activities. Consideration of the client's home care needs must cover a 24-hour period so the focus of direct care in home care nursing integrates the client, family, and any other caregivers that might be involved in providing direct care. Since home care is provided on a short-term, intermittent basis, the home care nurse's direct care always involves the client and caregivers so that care can be provided while the nurse is not present.

The home care nurse develops the care plan considering short- and long-term goals, which again takes into consideration the need to instruct the client, family, and caregiver to assume responsibility for learning the procedures, medications, and other aspects of the client's care plan. Third-party payors, such as Medicare, expect that the home care nurse will identify a competent caregiver for the client and instruct them on the client's care. Not only does this approach assure comprehensive coverage of the client's needs, but it can significantly decrease the number of home care visits that need to be done by home health agency personnel, resulting in lower costs. For example, after the home care nurse taught a spouse to do daily care for a peripheral vascular ulcer, daily nursing visits were decreased to twice weekly. The focus of the nurse's visits went from directly doing the procedure daily to seeing the client biweekly and (1) determining the extent of wound healing, (2) assessing for signs and symptoms of infection, (3) determining if the procedure was being completed appropriately, and (4) coordinating and communicating questions and progress reports with the client's primary physician.

The home care nurse is not routinely involved in the client's personal care, such as bathing, hair washing, or changing linen. Although these activities are essential to the client's recovery, if the client needs assistance with these beyond what the family may give, these tasks can be accomplished by a home health aide. This is not to say that the home care nurse should never get involved in the personal care of clients. During the course of a home visit you may be in a situation that requires you to bathe a client or help him change his clothing. You should perform these duties so that you can move on to provide the skilled nursing activities related to his direct care and that are the purpose of your home visit. If you find that every time you visit a particular client, there is a question of his receiving adequate personal care, you should evaluate the client's needs for the services of a home health aide or, if he has one, if there needs to be an increase in the amount of time the aide spends with him. You will also want to discuss your observations with the client's caregiver and determine strategies that will assist him or her in caring for the client. You may determine that the client needs more care than the family/caregiver are able to provide. In this instance, you would want to discuss other options, such as nursing home care, daycare, or other structured living arrangements.

Coordinating Services

In addition to providing direct care, the home care nurse is also responsible for the coordination of other professional and paraprofessional services involved in the client's care, even if not all these services are directly provided by the home health agency. Central to the role of coordinator of care is the ability to assess the client's needs, set priorities regarding problems that affect the recovery and independence of the client, identify how and if those needs can realistically be met, and develop a plan of action that can meet these needs. Also, the home care nurse is the main contact with the client's physician, both reporting pertinent changes in the client's condition and securing needed changes in the plan of care (Caring, 1988).

Referral to Other Resources. To function as a coordinator of services, you must be knowledgeable about the services offered by your own agency and the many resources available in the community. It is important that you have a clear understanding of the roles of other providers within your agency (PT, ST, OT, SW, HHA), and as part of your orientation program you should spend some time with these other people to learn more about their roles and functions and how you can work with them. You must also have a working knowledge about the services provided by those community resources outside your agency.

A community resource is any agency, organization, program, or service that delivers a service to residents of your community. The American Cancer Society, American Heart Association, American Red Cross, and Meals on Wheels are some of the well known community resources with which you might work. There are usually many more resources, depending on the size of your community and the specific needs of your clients. Your agency should have a list of often-used community resources and an explanation of the services they provide. Another community resource information source is the Yellow Pages of your telephone book. In your community there may also be an organization whose responsibility it is to coordinate and assure easy access to these resources for professionals and consumers. Talk with your supervisor about what is available in your area.

As you explore your community, it is helpful to keep the information you gain about each resource on a 3 × 5 index card and keep these in a small box. In this way, you begin a resource file that will be very helpful in your future work with various clients. Figure 2–2 provides an outline for recording information about a community resource. Use this to gather the information for your 3 × 5 cards.

Case Conferences. As the client's care coordinator, the home care nurse must have up-to-date information regarding the services provided by all care givers in the home. The sharing of information among these various providers is a difficult but not impossible task and is accomplished through the use of a case conference. At regularly scheduled times, and also as needed on an informal or formal basis, the home care nurse and others involved in the client's care discuss the client's response to the treatment plan and develop modifications to future goals. For example, the home care nurse may chair a case conference about a 65-year-old woman with the diagnosis of a right-sided cerebrovascular accident (CVA). Present at the conference are the physical therapist, the speech therapist, and the home health aide coordinator. In

---

Name of Agency:

Contact Person/Administrator:

Address: Telephone Number:

Hours of Operation:

Services Provided:

Eligibility Requirements:

Cost of Service:

Figure 2–2. Community Resource Information

this meeting, the physical therapist shares her assessment that the client has progressed satisfactorily with gait training and that she is anticipating the client's discharge from physical therapy within the next 2 weeks. The speech therapist also feels that the client's speech has progressed so well that the 2-week discharge date is appropriate for her discipline also. The nurse, considering this information, plans that her diet teaching and ongoing cardiovascular assessment goals can be reached also in the next 2 weeks if the client's condition doesn't change. From the case conference it becomes clear that the client will be ready for discharge in 2 weeks and should be informed immediately so that plans can be made for the home health agency to discharge the client. Also, it is important for the client to understand that since the covered services for Medicare (nursing, PT, and ST) are going to be terminated in 2 weeks, the home health aide visits will also need to be discontinued and that the client/family will have to explore other health aide services, if necessary. All case conferences should be documented in the client's home care record.

Sometimes, case conferences can occur over the telephone, mainly with caregivers that are not directly affiliated with the agency. For example, a case conference between the home care nurse and the client's primary physician might occur via telephone following a client's last physician visit. This may be necessary in order to determine the results of the doctor's visit and to adjust any changes in the plan of care. If the client is receiving occupational therapy from another agency, the nurse would want to schedule a conference with the occupational therapist relating to the client's care and record the telephone conference in the record, adjusting the plan of care appropriately.

Determining Financial Coverage

A unique feature of home care nursing is that the nurse must be involved constantly in the reimbursement aspects of the client's care. When a patient is admitted to a hospital, most frequently the nurse does not know how the patient is paying for his hospitalization, and all financial concerns are given to the business office. In home care, the nurse must determine who is going to pay for the services from the first visit until the time of discharge.

At the initial assessment, the home care nurse determines the type of service needed based on her assessment and the physician's orders. Before that aspect of the initial plan is completed the home care nurse must also determine if the payment source (private insurance, Medicare, Medicaid) will cover the specific type(s) of care. The nurse must work with her supervisor, billing office staff, the physician, and other care and service providers, if ordered, to develop the plan of care and discuss with the client what is and is not covered by payors. This is especially important since, if some services are not covered, the nurse must talk with the client and family to determine how other services needed or desired by the client are to be paid. This involvement with payment sources is very foreign to a nurse new to home care. Your agency should have a policy that deals with fee setting, specific forms to have clients sign relating to financial information, and procedures that outline who specifically is to handle various aspects of the financial plan for the clients' care. The section of Chapter 3 that deals with documentation outlines many of the restrictions and regulations involving financial coverage for home care services. Your agency should also have information about some payment sources that might be unique to your area.

Determining Duration of Care

Duration of care is defined as the amount and frequency of care given to a home care client. It is customary to determine the expected type and duration of care a client will receive after the initial home visit by all professional disciplines involved (Nsg., PT, ST, OT, SW), but nursing is usually the main service. Duration of care is determined by the home care nurse in collaboration with the client's physician, the agency supervisor, and the reimbursement source. Third party payors often have restrictions concerning the duration of care, which can be in the form of number of hours, number of visits, or dollars spent per specific period of time. For example, an insurance company may specify that only $500 can be spent on home care services per client per calendar year. The home care nurse, in collaboration with the client, must determine how to spend the money in the most efficient and effective manner that will still meet the client's needs. In some cases, the money could be spent on home health aide services, while in other situations it may be better spent on skilled nursing visits.

Medicare limits the duration of care by means of regulations placed on the client condition and type of home care services. In order for nursing services to be reimbursed by Medicare, the client must be acutely ill or experiencing an acute exacerbation of a chronic illness. Once the client becomes stable, Medicare will no longer cover home care services. This regulation often causes difficulty for elderly clients since many of them need services related to the many chronic illnesses they may have.

In some cases, a client doesn't have insurance coverage or has a policy that doesn't cover the needed care. Some agencies have a sliding fee scale so that a client, if eligible, can have care provided at a reduced fee. The home care nurse or some other member of the agency will work with the client/family to fill out a financial assessment form that lists the client's assets, income, and amount of debt. If the client is to receive a reduced fee, the agency can use this gathered information to determine how much the client can afford to pay for each visit. Ask your supervisor what your agency's policy is on a sliding fee scale.

In some areas, community agencies are able to assist with financing certain aspects of home care for those clients who are unable to pay. For example, the American Cancer Society will sometimes assist clients who have a terminal cancer diagnosis with the purchase of durable medical equipment (DME), such as a hospital bed. Other agencies in your community may have similar programs. This is another area in which learning about your community resources is essential to delivering quality home care services to your clients. This financial information is another item you can add to your community resources file.

Client Advocacy

Although the nurse's role as client advocate is not unique to home care, the way the nurse implements that role involves different knowledge and skills. When a home care nurse visits a client in the home following hospitalization, sometimes the most important issue for the client is how to access his insurance system so that he can pay the many bills that have accumulated due to his inpatient stay. Often these bills can be in a confusing format, without explanation of specific information, and can cause great anxiety in both client and family. Helping the client negotiate the complex system of health care insurance, or guiding him to someone who can, is an important advocacy role for the home care nurse. The stress caused by these financial matters prohibits the client from learning what he needs to know for the successful completion of his plan of care.

Again, community resource referral becomes an important advocacy role for the home care nurse. Clients may lack knowledge of the many community agencies that may be able to assist them. As the home care system grows, it becomes difficult for the professionals to keep informed of services. Imagine how complex the system appears for a lay person! Assisting the client and family in identifying community resources is an important role of the home care nurse.

At times, a referral to another health professional or organization may be necessary to provide the client with the most effective care. For example, if you find that a client is living in poverty and has many unpaid medical bills, the client may qualify for a state assistance program. In this case, you would make a referral to a social worker, either in your agency or one at the local assistance office, who can assist the client in the application process. Some clients and families will resist the idea of seeing a social worker, and it is up to you as their home care nurse to help them understand he or she is the professional with the skills needed to provide the proper care. Helping the client and family gain access to the most appropriate professional to meet their needs is another important advocacy role.

In summary, nurses in home care carry out a variety of roles and functions that build on traditional nursing skills. Providing direct care, coordinating care and services, determining financial coverage, determining duration of care, and being a client advocate are all unique challenges that home care nurses must meet to be successful. The next section will discuss the nursing process applied to home care and how it is similar to, yet very different from, institutional nursing practice.

NURSING PROCESS APPLIED TO HOME CARE

The nursing process is a framework that helps to organize and systematize the nursing care provided to clients. Home care nurses can use the steps of the nursing process as a guide to the practice of professional nursing in the home. The nursing process is a deliberative, problem-solving approach that requires technical, cognitive, and interpersonal skills and is directed toward meeting the client/family needs. These five steps of the nursing process

- Assessment
- Diagnosis
- Planning
- Implementation
- Evaluation

help the home care nurse to organize the nursing care to meet the specific needs of the client.

Using the nursing process benefits both the client and the family by encouraging their active participation in all phases of care. Also, continuity of care is assured through a systematic process of delivering care to clients. When the client care record is organized and completed according to the steps of the nursing process, the individualized care provided to the client is described clearly. This enhances communication between home care nurses, justifies coverage to third party payors, and allows the nurse and agency to document care that stands up legally and against standards and regulations.

The five steps of the nursing process are the same for all areas of practice. To review, the steps of the nursing process are:

Assessment involves activities that focus on gathering information regarding the client, the family, or the community for the purpose of identifying the client's needs, problems, or strengths. Using a systematic approach, data are collected through interview, physical assessment, and review of reports from other health care providers.

Diagnosis is the second phase of the nursing process. Nursing diagnosis involves the critical appraisal and analysis of the data collected during the assessment phase. It is during this phase that the nurse identifies the needs, problems, or strengths of the client which form the basis for the remainder of the nursing process.

Planning, the third phase of the nursing process, involves the development of strategies that will alter the identified problem or support the identified strength. In the planning phase, the needs, problems, or strengths identified are organized according to priority so that the one that is most significant to the client is cared for first. Less significant needs can be addressed after the primary need is met. Following the establishment of priorities, short- and long-term goals are identified, and nursing interventions are proposed that lead to the accomplishment of those goals.

Implementation is the fourth step of the nursing process and is defined as the initiation and completion of the designated activities that meet the goals outlined. In some cases, nurses may not be the exclusive providers of care during the implementation phase. The plan of care is used as a guide to the provider of care, whether the provider is the nurse, the client, or the family members. The implementation phase also includes recording the client care on the appropriate documents.

Evaluation is the fifth and final step of the nursing process. In this phase, the nurse determines which goals have been met and which goals have not yet been achieved. In collaboration with the client, the nurse tries to identify if goals continue to be realistic or need to be modified. If goals have not been achieved and continue to be important, perhaps a change in the plan of care to achieve the stated goals needs to be made. The identification of areas in the nursing care plan that require revision is an important part of this phase.

Although the nursing process is discussed as five distinct phases, it must be remembered that these phases, in practice, are very difficult to separate. The five phases of the nursing process are highly interdependent and interrelated. In the clinical setting, nurses are assessing the client's situation continually while at the same time they are developing some portions of the care plan and perhaps evaluating the attainment of other goals. The nursing process is also cyclical in nature. When you have completed the evaluation phase of the process, you often find that you need to go back to the assessment phase and collect more data so goals or interventions can be revised.

In home care, the nursing process is used as a framework or guide for providing care to the client. There are some unique characteristics that the nursing process assumes in the home care setting. In the following section each of the phases of the nursing process will again be discussed, this time with special attention to the application of the nursing process in the home setting.

Assessment

Assessment is described as the organized and systematic process of collecting data from a variety of sources to make a determination about the health status of a client (Iyer, Taptich, and Bernocchi-Losey, 1986). In home care, assessments are being made continually to update previously collected information or collect data in a totally new area. Much of the information about the client is collected during the admission visit, which is the first home visit made by the home care nurse. Some information about the client and his clinical problems may be gathered during the telephone call to the client and the initial intake information, but most of the data will be collected during the first home visit.

In planning for the first home visit, there are several areas that need to be considered. Supervisory staff at the agency usually have the responsibility of giving assignments of new cases to home care nurses. When given a new client, the home care nurse needs to review all the information about this client that is provided on the referral form or, if the client has been seen by the agency previously, an old record may be available. Although old records are sometimes very useful, a client's physiological or psychosocial status may have changed dramatically since he was last seen by the agency. Use the old record as a beginning point of assessment, recognizing the need to validate pertinent information and collect new data.

After you have reviewed all the information provided, you will want to make an initial telephone call to the client to arrange for the home visit. The initial contact between the home care nurse and the client is very important since it sets the stage for the relationship between the client and the agency. The home care nurse should identify herself and the employing agency clearly. For example, the nurse may say, "Hello Mr. Jones, this is Nancy Smith, a nurse from the VNA of Metropolis. You have been referred for home care from Metropolis Hospital, and I am calling to set up a visit for today." By identifying yourself,

your agency, and the way in which the client was referred to your agency, the client can feel assured that the call is legitimate and that there is a purpose for scheduling a visit.

When arranging for your first visit on the telephone there are certain issues you will want to address. First, you should be able to share with the client the purpose of the visit. Whether the client was referred to the agency for a procedure such as wound care, teaching, or monitoring, you can share the purpose of the visit with the client. In doing this, assessments can be made to determine if the client has sufficient supplies or equipment in the home to accomplish the designated task portion of the visit. For example, if the client needs wound care, you will want to ask him about the supplies he has in the home. Most home care agencies have a policy on the acquisition of supplies for the performance of a procedure in the home. Some agencies require the client's family to obtain the supplies necessary for the nurse to perform a specific procedure. In other agencies, the home care nurse assumes responsibility for ordering supplies and having them delivered before the home visit. You need to know your agency's policy with regard to obtaining supplies.

It is often helpful to arrange to have a significant other, such as a family member, with the client on this initial visit. If teaching needs to be done, the nurse can teach both the client and the family member at the same time. The home care nurse may also assess that a procedure such as wound care may be able to be done by a family member and teaching of this procedure can begin on this first visit. A family member is often instrumental in helping the home care nurse find needed items or operate such home appliances as the stove.

It is helpful for the home care nurse to ask a few other specific questions during this initial telephone encounter. These questions include

- What way will I be able to get into your home? (Front door, back door, first floor, door open or locked, etc.)
- Do you have any pets that will be a danger for a stranger entering your home?

Following the preliminary review of information and telephone call, the home care nurse is ready to make the initial visit to the client. It will be helpful if you arrive at the client's home close to the predetermined time. If you are unable to visit the client at the scheduled time, make every effort to call and reschedule. This shows the client that you recognize that he is a partner in his care and that his time is valuable. Clients will worry about your safety and the validity of the agency if communication is weak at the onset of care. Upon arrival at the client's home, you will spend the first few minutes of the visit in a social interaction with the client and his family. Introductions will be reinforced, and the tone will be set for this and future home visits.

Much of the structure for this initial home visit will be dictated by the initial visit procedure of your agency. Many agencies will provide the nurse with a patient care folder that includes many blank forms for the home care nurse to complete as part of the assessment process. These forms may include

- Physiological data base
- Psychosocial data base
- Financial data base
- Flow sheets, including a visit record
- Medication sheet
- Family roster
- Agency information, such as Bill of Rights, a brochure, or agency information, such as hours of operation, telephone numbers, or services provided

As these forms are filled out, the home care nurse should use all her senses to collect data to obtain a complete and accurate assessment of the client. The senses of smell, hearing, and touch may provide a wealth of information about the client, the family system of which he is a part, or the community in which he resides. For example, if you hear a great deal of arguing between family members during your home visit, you may question whether the client will be able to have a restful convalescence. Another situation may involve a client trying to recuperate from an exacerbation of emphysema in an industrial neighborhood with many pollutants in the air.

A complete and accurate assessment of the client includes data that is subjective, objective, current, and historical.

Objective data include the physical assessment and any other pieces of information observed or measured during the home visit. For example, objective data include such things as weight (176 pounds), blood pressure (126/46), or respiration rate (16).

Subjective data are the perceptions or view of the client about the situation. Subjective information may include statements the client makes regarding his prognosis or his perceptions regarding the reason he has a particular problem. Examples of subjective data include "I think I'm going to be all right now that I've had the surgery," or "I have this rash because of nerves."

Historical data are important to collect in order to establish a time frame for the current medical problem. Historical data involve information about the past medical history of the client and the significant behaviors that affected that past history.

Current data involve that information that is relevant to the medical problem the client is presently experiencing. Clients may have a tendency to spend a great deal of time telling the story of their past medical history. Although some of the information is useful, the home care nurse may need to channel the interview to the current medical problems to avoid lengthy and time-consuming interviews. This can be done through the use of such very specific questions as

- Can you tell me why you went into the hospital this time?
- What kind of diet were you on in the hospital?
- What happened just before you went into the hospital this time?

There are several methods of data collection the home care nurse must consider in the assessment stage. The three major methods of collecting data in the home are interviews, observation, and physical assessment. These three methods can be used together to provide the home care nurse with a full and accurate picture of the client situation.

Interviews involve asking well thought out, relevant, open-ended questions. The home care nurse may ask the client some questions while other questions may be directed towards the significant other. Since the purpose of the interview is to gather some of the subjective information needed to make a total assessment, it will be important for the nurse to be an active listener. Note taking during the interview will be helpful for charting following the interview, but remember, it is difficult to have an open, frank discussion with someone who is looking down at a piece of paper. Jot down key words and phrases that will help you to remember the important parts of the story. Try to maintain as much eye contact as possible to show the client that you are interested.

Direct observation will give you the most information about the client. In home care, the nurse observes not only the client's physical status and affect, but also the home, family relationships, and how the client is integrated into the family environment. Using all the senses, the home care nurse gathers significant information that will add to the total assessment of the client. For example, the home care nurse may go to a home for an initial visit to find the smell of alcohol permeating the house. One of the initial determinations that must be made is whether the client or some other member of the family is drinking. If the client is living with a significant other who is drinking, data may need to be gathered regarding the safety of the nurse and the client in that situation.

Physical examination is the third method of collecting data in this process, and involves physical assessment of the client to gather information about the physical status of the client, and validate subjective data gathered in the interviewing process. Many home care agencies will include a physical assessment form that can be used as a guide to collecting assessment information. Most approaches to physical assessment involve a head-to-toe assessment, using the techniques of inspection, palpation, percussion, and auscultation. If you are unsure about your physical assessment skills or need a refresher, there are many physical assessment texts and classes that may be helpful. You should discuss this with your supervisor.

In summary, much of the initial assessment of the client takes place during the first home visit. As the first step of the nursing process, assessment involves the collection of data about the client, his physical status, and the environment in which he lives. The home care nurse uses a variety of skills in the collection of data during the assessment process. These skills include interviewing, observation, and physical assessment. All these data collection strategies are useful in obtaining a full picture of the client.

Diagnosis

The next step in the nursing process involves the development of nursing diagnoses. A diagnosis is a statement of a problem or potential problem experienced by a client. The diagnosis stems logically from the data that are collected through the assessment process, and it mainly focuses on those areas that relate to independent nursing function. Independent nursing functions, those that do not require a physician's order, include such activities as teaching and assessment, and nursing interventions, such as turning, encouraging fluids, or reality orientation.

Nursing diagnosis is a relatively new phenomenon. In 1950, the term **nursing diagnosis** was introduced into the literature by Virginia Fry. At that time the American Nurses' Association did not support the concept. In the early 1970s, a group of nursing leaders recognized that nursing needed a method by which to label commonly seen health problems. In 1973 the first National Conference on the Classification of Nursing Diagnosis was held to begin to develop a list of accepted nursing diagnoses. This group has continued to meet annually to further refine the initial entries and develop a list that is inclusive of the types of problems nurses see in practice.

In 1982, the North American Nursing Diagnosis Association (NANDA) was developed from a task force of the 1973 conference. The North American Nursing Diagnosis Association (NANDA) became an integral force in the development and refinement of a system of nursing diagnoses in the United States. Also, they have been involved in promoting research in the area of nursing diagnosis and sharing the re-

sults of research and programs related to nursing diagnosis. NANDA publishes a list of approved nursing diagnoses, which can be used in clinical practice. The nursing diagnoses were developed using nine interactional patterns as the theoretical foundation. These interactional patterns, called *human response patterns*, are central to the care provided to clients by nurses. Figure 2–3 provides a list of the human response patterns that form the foundation of the diagnostic categories. This list now contains numerous diagnostic labels that have been approved for clinical use and testing. The NANDA list is included in Appendix 2 of this text.

There are many definitions of nursing diagnosis in professional literature. Many nurse practice acts suggest that nurses have the responsibility for diagnosing human responses to actual or potential problems of the client. Some early definitions of nursing diagnosis from the literature include

- Nursing diagnosis is a statement of a patient problem that is arrived at by making inferences from collected data. The problem is one that can be alleviated by nursing (Mundinger and Jauron, 1975).
- Nursing diagnoses made by professional nurses describe actual or potential health problems that nurses, by virtue of their education and experience, are capable and licensed to treat (Gordon, 1976).

For the purpose of this discussion, a nursing diagnosis is a statement of actual or potential health problems of a client that a nurse is legally able to treat. Whether the NANDA classification of identifying nursing diagnosis or another method is used, the purpose of writing nursing diagnoses is to communicate the client's problems to anyone who is reading the record. It also helps to organize the large volume of information that is collected during the assessment phase of the nursing process.

In some agencies, a classification system for writing nursing diagnosis is not used. Instead, nurses are asked to write nursing diagnoses of the client based on the information collected. A common method of

---

1. Exchanging—mutual giving and receiving
2. Communicating—sending messages
3. Relating—establishing bonds
4. Valuing—assigning relative worth
5. Choosing—selection of alternatives
6. Moving—activity
7. Perceiving—reception of information
8. Knowing—meaning associated with information
9. Feeling—subjective awareness of information

From McFarland, McFarlane, Nursing Diagnosis and Intervention. Philadelphia: C.V. Mosby Co., 1989.

Figure 2–3. Human response patterns

writing nursing diagnosis is the PES system. Using this method, the home care nurse identifies the **Problem, Etiology** and **Symptoms** of the client.

The first part of the diagnosis process, the problem, is defined as a short, concise statement of the client's health condition. For example, one problem experienced by a new diabetic may be lack of knowledge of foot care.

The second part of the nursing diagnosis is to determine the etiology. In this portion of the diagnosis, the factors that affect the existence of the problem are identified. Referring to the above example, lack of knowledge about foot care may be because the client, a newly diagnosed diabetic, has not yet attended any diabetic classes.

The third part of this diagnostic process relates to the signs or symptoms that provide evidence for the existence of the problem. Again using the previous example, the client's lack of knowledge about proper foot care may be determined by his expressions of a lack of knowledge and the home care nurse's observations of the client walking barefoot in the house. The following are additional examples of nursing diagnoses, written using the PES method.

- Difficulty with accomplishment of activities of daily living (ADLs) due to immobility from fractured hip, as evidenced by patient expression of difficulty and condition of house at time of home care nurse's visit
- Difficulty breathing due to exacerbation of chronic obstructive pulmonary disease (COPD), as evidenced by shallow noisy respirations, diaphoresis, and extreme fatigue
- Decubitus ulcer due to long-standing immobility and poor nutrition, as evidenced by 2″ × 2″ × 1″ wound on coccyx

In summary, the diagnosis phase of the nursing process is when the data collected in the assessment phase are processed and organized into meaningful statements so that planning can begin. In home care, accurate and complete nursing diagnoses are critical to efficient communication between home care nurses and to providing a means for problem identification, which is a necessary element for reimbursement.

Planning

The planning phase of the nursing process begins after the formulation of the nursing diagnosis and concludes with the documentation of the plan of care. Planning involves the development of strategies designed to prevent, minimize, or correct the problems identified in the nursing diagnosis. (Iyer, Taptich, and Bernocchi-Losey, 1986). The planning compo-

nent of the nursing process consists of four stages, which will be discussed individually. They are

- Setting priorities
- Writing goals
- Implementation strategies
- Documentation

Setting Priorities. There are many theoretical models that can be used to help the home care nurse develop priorities of care. One such model is Maslow's Hierarchy of Needs. Maslow's Hierarchy of Needs suggests that there are five levels of need experienced by man. These levels are physiological, safety or security, social, esteem, and self-actualization. Maslow suggests that the physiological needs must be met before the client may be willing or able to meet the higher level needs. For example, a home care nurse identifies two problems being experienced by the client, incontinence and social isolation. Maslow suggests that the physiological problem of incontinence should have a higher priority than the upper level problem of social isolation because once the physiological problem is addressed, the client will be better able to deal with that problem and the nurse can better assess and evaluate how the social isolation can be overcome.

Writing Goals. Following the identification of priorities of care, the home care nurse will develop goals or outcomes. Goals are statements defining specific behaviors that demonstrate that the problem has been corrected, minimized, or prevented (Iyer et al., 1986). They are derived from the nursing diagnoses identified in the previous phase of the nursing process. For example, if a nursing diagnosis identifies constipation as a problem for a specific client, the goals related to this diagnosis would identify the specific behaviors the client could demonstrate that would indicate that constipation was no longer a problem. In this case, a goal might be "The client will have a bowel movement within 1 day and every 3 days thereafter without straining." These statements will provide the mechanism for the evaluation of the effectiveness of the care provided.

Clearly written goals are essential to effective communication between home care nurses. Nurses unfamiliar with the client should be able to read the goals and understand what they mean. More importantly, the nursing staff member should be able to work toward this goal with the client when the primary nurse is unavailable. There are six rules or guidelines for developing meaningful and understandable goals (Iyer, Taptich, Bernocchi-Losey, 1986).

1. Goals should be client centered.

   Goals are always written in terms of what behaviors the nurse wants **the client** to achieve.

2. Goals should be clear and concise.

   Long, involved goals are frequently difficult to understand. In writing goals, try to use simple words and phrases with approved abbreviations.

3. Goals should be observable and measurable.

   In writing goals, the home care nurse is identifying what **the client** will do following the interventions. These behaviors must be observable and measurable so that it can be determined if the interventions were effective. Avoid goals that are too vague. For example, how can you measure a goal that states "the client will know about his COPD"? Can you observe or measure knowledge? This goal needs to be rewritten to reflect the measurable elements of the client's knowledge. These measurable elements may be
   - The client will identify three factors that cause difficulty breathing.
   - The client will list, in sequence, the steps he must take when short of breath.
   - The client will identify two safety measures associated with having oxygen in the home.

4. Goals should be time limited.

   A time frame for achievement of the goal should be clearly identified as part of the goal. Some goals will be achieved early in the care of the client, while others will be achieved by the time of discharge. A time frame allows the home care nurse to evaluate the necessity of certain nursing diagnoses as goals are met.

5. Goals should be realistic.

   In writing goals in the home care setting, the nurse must take into account both the resources of the client and the home environment. It would be unrealistic for the home care nurse to write a goal that "the client will obtain a maid service to clean up the home environment" for a client living in poverty. A more realistic goal in this situation might be "within the next 2 days, the client will request help from his two children to clean up his home."

6. Goals should be mutually agreeable between the client and the nurse.

   Goals should not be written by the home care nurse in isolation. Following the identification of nursing diagnoses, the home care nurse and the client discuss the behaviors that will be achieved as a result of the interventions being specified. Contracting is a strategy that can be effective in determining goals and the methods to achieve them. This active participation between the nurse and the client allows for the validation of expectations and the sharing of unrealistic perceptions before the care plan is instituted.

Implementation Strategies

Implementation strategies are those activities carried out with the purpose of helping the client achieve the identified goals. These activities are clearly defined approaches for meeting the client's goals. By documenting clearly the interventions that must be done, the nurse can avoid the need for long, drawn out reports when someone unfamiliar with the case needs to fill in and see the client. In addition to the specific strategy, the home care nurse needs to consider *who* will work with the client on the identified strategy.

Some activities will be carried out exclusively by the nurse. For example, biweekly blood pressure assessment is an intervention done by the home care nurse. The home care nurse may assign certain responsibilities to the paraprofessionals in the agency, such as the home health aide. If a goal for a client was to have a weekly bath and the client was unable to accomplish this, a home health aide might be assigned to the case to help the client meet this goal. It must be remembered that although the home health aide has the responsibility for giving the client the bath, the home care nurse retains responsibility for all aspects of the client's care. Regular supervisory visits are indicated to assure that the goals are being met through the use of the home health aide.

Other intervention strategies are carried out exclusively by the client. An example of this might be the client who takes full responsibility for insulin self-administration following instruction by the home care nurse. In some instances, the client and the home care nurse share responsibility for an intervention. An example of this might be when a home care nurse performs wound care on Tuesday and Friday while the client performs wound care on the rest of the days of the week. This arrangement is very useful in that it allows the nurse to assess the healing of the wound while the client maintains primary responsibility for the care of the wound. This can be a valuable approach for teaching the client wound care.

How does the home care nurse determine what interventions are appropriate for a particular client? It is most helpful to begin with the medical diagnosis furnished by the hospital and physician. There are certain interventions to be done for every client with a specific diagnosis. For example, an assessment of a client's peripheral vascular status and inspection of the feet are indicated for every diabetic. Similarly, for every cardiac client, assessment of the blood pressure and pulse would be performed on each visit. Some agencies provide flow sheets for specific illnesses or conditions that detail the basic interventions for a client with the identified illness. These are very useful in identifying the common interventions for all clients with a specific illness. You may want to see if your agency uses standardized flow sheets. The use of flow sheets will be discussed in Chapter 3, which covers documentation.

Other sources of information that can be useful to the home care nurse in developing the interventions for the client are the many books of standard care plans written for home care clients. These texts take a specific diagnosis, nursing or medical, and suggest interventions for the care of a client with that particular diagnosis. Again, these texts present the interventions generally so that they may be applicable to all clients with the identified diagnosis. An example of a standard care plan can be found in Appendix 3.

Since both flow sheets and standard care plans are generic in nature, that is they do not take into account the unique needs of a particular client, the interventions must be personalized to reflect the needs and characteristics of the client and his environment. The home care nurse identifies the unique characteristics of the client during the assessment phase of the nursing process, and these characteristics should be integrated into the care plan. For example, a home care nurse finds out that the client being admitted to the agency has worked for 45 years on the night shift in a local factory. He has just been discharged from the hospital on a regime of insulin—24 units of NPH every AM. Based on the standard care plan for this client, the home care nurse would teach the client to give himself insulin at 7:30 AM. Your initial assessment reveals that the regular sleep pattern for this client is a 3:00 AM bedtime with a 10:00 awakening. In this case, the home care nurse would design a personalized care plan and have the client self-administer the insulin at 11:00 AM.

The home care nurse uses the home visit as the mechanism for accomplishment of many of the identified strategies or interventions. The home visit is the single most important tool of the home care nurse. It is through the visit process that the nurse gains insight into the client's health and life-style. This information is essential in planning and implementing appropriate intervention strategies. More about the specific nature and components of the home visit are found in the next section.

Evaluation

Although evaluation is one of the most significant steps in the care of clients, it is often neglected or incompletely done. Evaluation is defined as the planned, systematic comparison of the client's health status with the objectives that were identified in the planning phase. The use of the agreed upon goals is essential to the evaluation process.

Evaluation is discussed as the final phase of the nursing process, but in fact, some evaluation is occurring during all phases of the nursing process. The evaluation that occurs regularly throughout all phases of the nursing process is called *formative evaluation*. The home care nurse will need to evaluate the care given regularly throughout the client's interaction with the agency. For example, a home care nurse and client may mutually agree that a goal of care is "the client will be able to perform independent wound care after three teaching sessions." Following the first teaching session, the home care nurse needs to evaluate if all the planned material for that teaching session was covered. If not, perhaps the objective needs to be altered at this point rather than waiting until the three sessions are completed. Following the first teaching session, the nurse may determine that the client had difficulty understanding the teaching that was done. Perhaps the client had difficulty performing the psychomotor skills necessary to meet the objective. It may even be that the client originally thought he could perform the dressing change but when required to do so, he felt squeamish about the procedure. Whatever the reason, the home care nurse needs to modify the objective to fit the needs and abilities of the client.

Evaluation done in the final stages of the client–nurse relationship is called **summative evaluation**. This type of evaluation occurs when the client is getting ready to be discharged from the agency. Again, the home care nurse will evaluate the client's achievement of the identified goals. At the time of discharge from the agency it is hoped that the client will have satisfactorily achieved the goals agreed upon in an earlier phase of the interaction. Achievement of goals is an indication that the client can be discharged from home care services.

When evaluating the effectiveness of the care plan, the home care nurse may find that there was not complete or adequate achievement of the goals. The reasons for this may not be obvious to either the nurse or the client. There are several questions the nurse can ask in the process of examining why client goals have not been achieved.

- Did I have enough information about the client and his problem to develop goals appropriately?
- Were the goals realistic for this client?
- Was there some factor outside the client's control

(e.g., family dynamic, housing problem) that made it impossible for him to achieve the goal?

- Were the goals mutually agreed upon or were they developed exclusively by the nurse?
- Did the client have other priorities that prevented him from focusing on the identified problem and goal?
- Was the problem perceived by the client, and did the client feel that resolution of the problem was a priority?
- Were the intervention strategies appropriate?
- Did the family have the resources (e.g., financial, transportation) to meet the goals?
- If other health care providers were involved in the care, was there coordination of care to facilitate the achievement of the goal?

The use of evaluation helps the home care nurse provide care that is designed to meet the needs of the client in a cost effective and efficient manner. It also helps the nurse to modify goals and interventions as the need arises over the course of the interaction with the client. Evaluation also helps the home care nurse determine when the client can be discharged from home care services.

To summarize, the nursing process is a method of collecting and organizing information so that nursing care can be implemented to meet the identified needs of the client. The nursing process consists of five steps: assessment, diagnosis, planning, implementation, and evaluation. Benefits of using the nursing process in home care include enhanced communication between home care nurses, clearer justification for reimbursement for third party payors, and the development of a care plan that is designed to meet the needs of the client.

INFECTION CONTROL IN HOME CARE

As part of your preparation for home visiting, you need to consider the type of client you are going to visit. Recent trends in medical care have resulted in increasingly ill clients being cared for in the home. As hospital stays have shortened, clients with communicable diseases and multiple invasive devices are now being cared for in the home by the home care nurse. There are two major concerns for the home care nurse in caring for these clients. They are

1. How to prevent infection in clients who are debilitated and may be immunocompromised
2. How to protect the nurse, family, and community from a client who has an infectious or communicable disease

The home setting provides some special challenges for the home care nurse in preventing the spread of infection or protecting the immunocompromised client from pathogens. For example, the primary caregivers, usually family members, are often untrained in procedures and know little about aseptic technique. The home may also lack the facilities to care for the client under optimal conditions. In some homes, there may not be access to running water, a heating unit to boil equipment, or adequate facilities to dispose of contaminated equipment. The unique nature of the home as the setting for care necessitates the development of unique solutions to the problems encountered by the home care nurse. To address this, agencies have developed policies and procedures that deal with infection control, usually based on procedures developed nationally.

Universal Blood and Body Fluid Precautions

The Centers for Disease Control (CDC) recommends the use of universal blood and body fluid precautions by all home health professionals for all patients regardless of the diagnosis. Since medical history or physical examination cannot reliably identify all patients infected with a bloodborne pathogen, blood and body fluid precautions should be used consistently to protect the health care worker from acquiring an infectious disease. Universal blood and body fluid precautions described by the CDC are detailed in Table 2–1.

Universal precautions apply to blood and to other body fluids containing visible blood. Universal precautions also apply to other body fluids, including semen, vaginal secretions, cerebrospinal fluid, synovial fluid, pleural fluid, peritoneal fluid, pericardial fluid, and amniotic fluid. Universal precautions do not apply to feces, nasal secretions, sputum, sweat, tears, urine, saliva, and vomitus, unless they contain visible blood. Although the use of gloves may not be mandated when dealing with such body fluids as saliva, the home care nurse needs to use the general infection control practices already in existence. For example, gloves may be indicated during digital examination of the oral mucosa or during endotracheal suctioning, and handwashing is necessary following the exposure to saliva. Gloves need not be worn when feeding patients or wiping saliva from the skin (Morbidity and Mortality Weekly Report [MMWR], 1988).

Human breast milk has been implicated in the perinatal transmission of human immunodeficiency virus (HIV) but has never been implicated in the transmission of HIV or Hepatitus B virus (HBV) to health care workers. The health care workers do not

TABLE 2–1. UNIVERSAL BLOOD AND BODY FLUID PRECAUTIONS

The following is a general description of universal blood and body fluid precautions, as described by the CDC for use by all health care workers (MMWR, 1988).

1) All health care workers should routinely use appropriate barrier precautions to prevent skin and mucous membrane exposure when contact with blood or other body fluids of any patient is anticipated. Gloves should be worn for touching blood or body fluids, mucous membranes, or non-intact skin of all patients; for handling items or surfaces soiled with blood or body fluids; and for performing venipuncture and other vascular access procedures.

2) Hands and other skin surfaces should be washed immediately and thoroughly if contaminated with blood or other body fluids. Hands should be washed immediately after gloves are removed.

3) All health care workers should take precautions to avoid injuries caused by needles, scalpels, and other sharp devices during procedures; during disposal of used equipment such as needles; when cleaning used equipment; and when handling sharp instruments after procedures. To prevent needlestick injuries, needles should not be recapped, purposefully bent or broken by hand, or removed from disposable syringes. After they are used, sharp instruments should be placed in a puncture proof container for disposal.

4) Although saliva has not been implicated in human immunodeficiency virus (HIV) transmission, to minimize the need for emergency mouth-to-mouth resuscitation, mouthpieces should be available for use.

5) Health care workers who have exudative lesions or weeping dermatitis should refrain from all direct patient care and from handling patient care equipment until the condition resolves.

6) Pregnant health care workers are not known to be at greater risk of contracting HIV infections than other health care workers who are not pregnant; however, if a health care worker develops HIV infection during pregnancy, the infant is at risk of infection resulting from perinatal transmission. Because of this risk, pregnant health care workers should be especially familiar with and adhere strictly to precautions to minimize the risk of HIV infection.

From Morbidity and Mortality Weekly Report, *(1988), with permission.*

have intensive exposure to breast milk as does the nursing neonate. Although universal precautions do not apply to human breast milk, gloves may be worn by health care workers who are frequently exposed to breast milk. Gloves should always be worn in situations when the breast milk is contaminated with visible blood.

If your agency does not provide each home care nurse with a puncture proof container, you may want to carry a baby bottle with you for the disposal of needles. When you have used a needle during the home visit, you can place the uncapped needle directly in the baby bottle, cap the bottle and transport it safely to your agency where there is a puncture proof container. The baby bottle can be uncapped and tipped to allow the needle to fall into the puncture proof container without the nurse having to touch the used needle.*

Your agency will have a procedure regarding the use of universal precautions in the care of clients in the home. You should review this procedure carefully, making yourself familiar with the steps you must take when providing direct care to clients. Although it may seem simple, handwashing is an important activity the home care nurse can perform to remove from the hands the disease-producing organisms and viruses acquired from direct contact with the client. If possible, handwashing should be done using soap and running water for at least 10 seconds.

It is always a good idea for the home care nurse to carry in the nursing bag a handwashing agent, such as an alcohol foam or antiseptic rinse, that does not require running water (Scott, Trusler, and Simmons, 1988). Table 2–2 is a review of universal precautions do's and don'ts.

Measures to Control the Spread of Communicable Disease

The presence of a family member with a communicable disease in the home need not be a health hazard to other members of the household or the community in which he resides. There may be many misconceptions, based on fear, about the care of the client with an infectious disease and the spread of the disease to members of the household. The home care nurse can be instrumental in providing answers to questions and allaying the fears of the family caregivers.

The isolation precautions in the home should be based on common sense, practicality, and knowledge of disease transmission. The following are guidelines that can be used in the home to control the spread of communicable disease (Berg, 1988).

1. The most appropriate and effective method of disease prevention is handwashing.
2. Excessive isolation practices in the home, in addition to being impractical and inappropriate, may compromise the quality of patient care in the home and socially isolate the client.

---

*This suggestion was given to the authors by Diane St. Pierre-Masten, VNA of the Berkshires.

TABLE 2–2. UNIVERSAL PRECAUTIONS, DO'S AND DONT'S

- DO wash your hands thoroughly with soap, running water, and friction before and immediately after patient contact, between patients, and after removing gloves. Wash hands immediately after contact with blood or any body fluids that apply to universal precautions.
- DO wear gloves when handling contaminated articles, such as dressings, linen, and lab specimens.
- DO wear gowns, masks, or goggles, as well as gloves, to protect yourself during procedures that may involve splashing of blood or contaminated body fluids.
- DO wear gloves if you have minor cuts, scratches, or inflammation on your hands.
- DO prevent injuries from needles, scalpels, and other sharp instruments.
- DO wear gloves when coming in contact with blood, body fluids containing visible blood, and other body fluids to which universal precautions apply.
- DON'T recap, bend, or break used needles.
- DO place used disposable syringes, needles, and sharp items into a puncture resistant container.
- DON'T disregard an accidental needlestick or other exposure, such as a splash to the eyes or mouth.
- DO cleanse the site thoroughly with soap and water and contact your supervisor immediately.
- DO dispose of articles (used dressings, gloves, bandages, etc.) contaminated with blood or body fluids into a plastic bag. Close the bag tightly, place it into a second plastic bag, and discard bag into a plastic-lined trash can.
- DO treat all linen and clothing soiled with blood or body fluids (to which universal precautions apply) as infectious.
- DO wear gloves and gown when removing such linen or clothing.
- DO place the soiled articles into a plastic bag and later wash the articles in hot water (160°) with detergent for 25 minutes.
- DO clean all blood and body fluid spills promptly. Use detergent and water followed by a disinfectant solution of one part household bleach to ten parts water.

3. Client wastes (feces, urine, blood, contents of suction canisters, etc.) can be flushed safely down the toilet. Waste matter of AIDS clients can be disposed of in the same manner and does not need special treatment.

4. Disposable dishes are not indicated for home care clients with infectious diseases. The client's dishes and eating utensils can be washed, along with the family dishes, in hot, soapy water or washed in the family dishwater on the hot cycle.

5. Sharing personal articles (e.g., combs, razors, towels, toothbrushes) between client and family members should be avoided.

6. Clients and caregivers should be educated to use gloves when changing the dressings of infected or draining wounds. The importance of handwashing, even though gloves are worn, must be emphasized.

7. Soiled dressings, used gloves, disposable equipment, and so forth should be saturated with bleach, placed in plastic bags, tied, and discarded in the trash can. This method is also appropriate for discarding patient care items used for AIDS clients.

8. Soiled linens and clothing (including those used by AIDS clients) can be laundered in the family washer using the hot cycle, detergent, and one cup of bleach and dried in the family dryer on the hot cycle.

9. Blood spills and other body secretion spills should be cleaned with a good household disinfectant (e.g., alcohol, peroxide, bleach, or Lysol, diluted as directed). Gloves should be worn to protect skin from disinfectant and body fluids.

10. Home clients with enteric disease should not be allowed to assist in food preparation until symptoms resolve or results from two consecutive cultures taken at least 24 hours apart are negative. The client should practice scrupulous handwashing at all times. If it is not possible to exclude the patient from food preparation (e.g., a single mother of two small children), the client must be educated to practice strict handwashing and hygiene during food preparation.

11. Clients with enteric infections do not require a private bathroom if they practice good hygiene. If the client is unable to practice good hygiene, a private bathroom should be considered. (Note: In homes with one or no bathroom, the best approach is to clean fecal contamination immediately with a household disinfectant.)

12. Clients with respiratory infections should be instructed to cover all coughs and sneezes with a tissue and discard the tissue in a designated receptacle. Clients should also wash their hands after coughing and sneezing.

Measures for the Immunocompromised Client

The immunocompromised client is often seen in the home care setting. The inability of a client to resist infection can be the result of many conditions (AIDS, bone marrow suppression from chemotherapy, a side effect of other pharmacological agents, etc.) and poses unique challenges to the home care nurse. For the client who is immunocompromised, there are special precautions that must be taken to avoid the development of infectious diseases. These precautions include

1. Avoid contact with family members or visitors who have a contagious disease (Berg, 1988).
2. Avoid raw foods, such as salads, raw eggs (as in egg nog), and unpasteurized milk (Berg, 1988).
3. Use precautions when caring for pets. Avoid emptying litter boxes, cleaning bird cages, and aquariums (Berg, 1988).
4. Use small containers for food, and use contents completely at one serving to prevent leftovers (Humphrey, 1986).
5. Provide clients with their own eating utensils, dishes, and glasses (Humphrey, 1986).
6. Avoid cut flowers and houseplants. Water standing in containers for long periods of time is a medium for bacteria growth (Humphrey, 1986).

The prevention of the spread of a communicable disease can be accomplished when the caregivers and the home care nurse fully understand the principles of care involved and continue to use proper technique. Caring for a client with an infectious disease in the home need not be a danger for other members of the household or the community in which the client resides. Clients, caregivers, and home care nurses can work together to make the care safe and humanistic.

HOW TO DO A HOME VISIT

Overall Considerations

The home visit is the most frequent way the home care nurse provides care to clients. Steps of the home visit will be discussed in this section. Learning to conduct a home visit using these steps makes the implementation of the home visit easier. At first, home visiting will seem cumbersome and difficult since a great deal of planning must go into a visit so it can be completed in an efficient and effective manner. As you make more home visits, your proficiency will increase, and the planning and implementation time for visits will decrease.

Home visiting is significantly different from providing care to patients in the hospital. The most obvious difference is the environment itself. In the hospital or outpatient clinic setting, the environment is controlled by the health care provider. In the home setting, the environment is controlled by the client and the family. In the home, the home care nurse does not have the immediate support of colleagues

and the sophisticated structure of a hospital to assist in the provision of care. The nurse is seen as a guest in the client's home, a home that often is ill-suited to the provision of care. There may be no running water or telephone, or the house may be in a state of disrepair. The home care nurse must recognize these values and norms and accept the client's living situation, even though it may be very different than one to which she is accustomed. By working through these values, the home care nurse will be a more effective provider of care.

There are other considerations of being a guest in the client's home. For example, be careful not to track mud or snow in to the client's home as you enter. If your feet do become dirty before you enter the home, tell the client this and ask where you may wipe them off. Always ask permission to wash your hands before starting the care for the client.These kindnesses show respect and consideration for the client and family and set up your relationship as nonthreatening.

Since the home visit provides the home care nurse with the opportunity to see the client in his home environment, the nurse may see the client surrounded by familiar things and be able to assess his cultural beliefs and traditions. Home visits also allow the nurse to observe the client/family system, which is essential for planning and implementing nursing care. During the home visit, behaviors and values, which provide insights into the family structure and function, can be observed. For example, the home care nurse may observe relationships with pets, the assignment of family roles and tasks, decor and orderliness of the home, the character of the interactions between family members (e.g., boisterous, timid, angry, or compassionate), the value placed on privacy, and many other variables that affect the client's care. This is why the home visit is seen as the single most important tool of the home care nurse.

Since the home is often not set up specifically for the care of the sick member, there may be times when you have to rearrange small pieces of furniture or items on a table. Before doing this, ask the client or family if it would be all right if, for example, you could move the trinkets on a night table so you could set up your dressing materials. Most families are more than willing to make the necessary accommodations to the home care nurse's needs. When you are finished with the procedure, always offer to replace all the rearranged items. If the procedure must be performed on a regular basis, you may want to encourage the family to find other places for the items until the area is no longer needed for the procedure. Always give the family the option of returning all items to their original position when you leave.

Personal Safety. There are certain safety factors all nurses who make home visits must take into consideration. While it is rare that the personal safety of the nurse is compromised, the nurse's safety is a prime concern before, during, and after the home visit. If you feel there exists a potentially unsafe situation, discuss this with your supervisor before making the home visit. If you are concerned about your safety while in the home, leave, and discuss this matter with your supervisor. Some agencies have an escort system, and many have specified policies and procedures concerning safety in certain agency service areas. Discuss this with your supervisor and review any policies available.

Safety Tips. There are some safety tips the home care nurse can employ during various stages of the home visit.

- Know where you are going and how to get there. Use a map for directions. There should be a section on the client's home care record indicating specific directions.
- Avoid carrying a purse or pocketbook. Have some change and your identification in your pocket. Lock your pocketbook in the trunk of your car before you leave the agency.
- Park as close to the client's home as possible. Know how you will gain access to the client's home or apartment. Lock your car doors.
- Dress appropriately and within the guidelines established by the agency. Wear comfortable shoes, ones that you can run in, if necessary.
- In the home, if you have fears about your safety, if people in the home are drunk, or there are weapons evident, do what is necessary, if you can, and then leave. If you feel you must leave immediately, do so.
- If pets are bothersome during the home visit, insist that they be put in another room. Some pets may become hostile as you begin to work with a client since they may perceive that you are harming their master.
- Avoid walking down alleys or on private property to take a shortcut to or from a client's residence. Carry a flashlight for poorly lit corridors. If you are unsure about a corridor or hallway leading to a client's home, ask a family member to meet you at the entrance to the building and show you the way.
- Know the telephone numbers of your agency, the local police, and the fire department. Know the policy for emergencies at your agency.
- Keep your nursing bag within your sight. When you are not using it, keep it closed and latched. This will protect it from curious pets and children and reduce the possibility of having unwanted pests enter the bag.
- Never walk into a home uninvited. Always knock and be assured verbally that someone is home before entering, even when the client has left the door unlocked for you.

Home Visiting Steps

Steps of the home visit are broken down into three stages, each with activities that must be accomplished before another stage is begun. The three stages are

1) the pre-visit stage
2) the visit stage
3) the post-visit stage

Each stage will be described and discussed in this section. The stages of the home visit, with specific activities, are summarized in Figure 2–4.

The Pre-Visit Stage. The pre-visit stage includes activities that prepare the home care nurse to accomplish the tasks of the home visit. The first step of this stage is to familiarize yourself with the client's chart and the purpose of your home visit. This is helpful in planning your day since some clients will require visits at specific times, and some visits take longer than others. For example, if the chart indicates that the purpose of the home visit is to observe the client administer her morning insulin, clearly the home care nurse needs to be at the client's home early in the morning. In some cases, clients have sophisticated and complex procedures that need to be done. By

---

Pre-visit activities
Familiarize yourself with the client's chart
Telephone call to the client to confirm visit and time
Thorough review of the client's chart
Arrange necessary equipment for the visit
Review the route to the client's home
Leave schedule for the day at the agency

Visit activities
Social phase (brief)
Wash hands and arrange equipment
Implement activities of care plan
Gather equipment and wash hands
Plan for next home visit

Post-visit activities
Revise care plan, if needed
Documentation
Communication with members of the health care team
Referrals, if indicated
Care for used equipment
Replenish nursing bag

Figure 2–4. The Home Visiting Process

reviewing the chart, the home care nurse can plan to spend the needed time with the client.

An important pre-visit activity is the telephone call to the client to confirm the visit. In most cases of follow-up visits, the home care nurse has planned with the client at the previous visit when subsequent visits will be made. Even though this may have been done previously, it is essential that the client be called to confirm that he is expecting a visit and that the time of the visit is convenient. This telephone call should be brief, but it is useful to ask the client how he or she is feeling and if there has been a significant change in the client's condition since the last home visit. Avoid allowing the client to go into a long description of all his or her health problems, and tell him or her that you will be there shortly to discuss it. If there has been a change in the client's condition, you can plan for this visit more easily before leaving the office. Perhaps you will need to review some books to determine the proper assessment or intervention, or perhaps a case conference with your supervisor is indicated.

Once the home visit is planned and confirmed by the telephone call, a thorough review of the chart takes place. You need to be thoroughly familiar with the client's history, medical problems, medication regime, and care plan with special attention given to the client's specific interventions. Your supervisor or another nurse may be instrumental in filling you in on some aspects of the case, but a thorough review of the chart should provide you with the information you need. (This makes a strong case for good documentation!) From this review, you can plan the agenda of your visit. If you are unfamiliar with a medication or specific intervention, go to a nursing text. Before entering the client's home you should have a mental picture of how the visit will unfold, but always remain flexible since priorities and clients' needs change and this affects the course of the home visit.

The next pre-visit activity is checking your nursing bag and arranging the necessary equipment. If your agency uses nursing bags, it is your responsibility for keeping the bag well stocked and in good condition. There are certain items basic to all nursing bags, and they are listed in Figure 2–5. Since you have reviewed the interventions that need to be accomplished, additional necessary equipment can be easily assembled. For example, if you know that a blood sugar is needed for Mr. Brown as part of his care plan, you must plan to do a blood test on this visit and take a glucometer with you.

Before you leave the agency, the route to the client's home should be reviewed. You should always carry a map, but if the map is reviewed in the agency

Soap
Paper towels
Forceps
Scissors
Thermometers (oral and rectal)
Cotton balls
Tongue depressors
4 × 4 gauze
Gauze
Gloves—clean (ample supply)
Sterile gloves (one pair)
Apron
Syringe—needles (assorted lengths and gauges)
Tape
Alcohol wipes
Tape measure
Flashlight
Stethoscope and sphygmomanometer
Map
Copy of *Home Care Nursing*

*This is a list of the standard equipment that is part of all home care nursing bags. Your agency may have additional items that nurses are required to carry and that may need special standing orders (e.g., adrenaline).

Figure 2–5. The Contents of the Nursing Bag*

and directions are written out, the chances of getting lost are reduced. If it is important that directions to the client's home be written on the record on admission. If this is done consistently, subsequent visits are easier and quicker.

You will need to leave your proposed daily schedule at the agency so you may be reached while you're out. Some agencies use a tickler system that consists of a small box and 3 × 5 cards, each with the name of a client on it. The tickler box is divided with index cards for each day of the month. As the nurse sees a client, the index card is filed behind the index card for the date of the next scheduled home visit. In this way, clients don't get lost and the scheduled visits for a specific day are easy to identify. Other agencies ask the nurses to fill out a route slip with the client's name and anticipated visit time. Many agencies use computers to assist with this function. This activity is more important than it may seem. Sometimes a client will call the agency to cancel a visit or a physician will call with new orders after a nurse has left for the day. By knowing where the nurse is, the supervisor can call the preceding patient and leave that message. On a more personal note, you may need to be reached while in the field for a personal emergency, so if care is taken with your schedule the supervisor will have little difficulty reaching you.

The Visit Stage. The initial face-to-face meeting between the nurse and the client is very important since it sets the tone for the relationship to follow. The first few minutes of the home visit are generally viewed as the social phase, when the client and the home care nurse may have some light conversation so that both are put at ease. After this phase, the nurse is ready to begin to implement the care plan. As discussed before, the equipment you need on the home visit will usually be carried in your nursing bag. Although "bag technique" is often thought of as an old fashioned concept, it is an important part of asepsis in the home. Techniques for the use and care of the nursing bag are essential to reduce the spread of organisms from one client to another, from nurse to client, or from client to nurse. The following steps in bag technique should be used on every visit to maximize the efficient and effective use of the nursing bag.

Bag Technique

1. Place the bag in a clean area, preferably on a wooden table. If a clean area cannot be found, the bag should always be placed on something like a newspaper to avoid contaminating the outside of the bag. Do not place your bag on stuffed furniture or at a level where an inquisitive child or pet can gain access to the bag and contaminate it or harm themselves. Always keep your bag in sight.
2. Select something that will be used to discard contaminated equipment, such as a paper or plastic bag, or a bag made from newspaper.
3. Wash your hands using the soap and paper towels in your bag. It is always best to use your own soap and towels unless the patient has paper towels for your use. Do not use a cloth towel unless the patient has one for your use only. Leave the equipment at the sink until the end of the visit.
4. Only now, after handwashing, can the nurse enter the bag and take out the equipment needed for the visit. Place the equipment on a clean paper towel.
5. Proceed with the visit and discard dirty equipment into the paper or plastic bag. If syringes are used, you should know the agency's procedure for discarding them. Check this procedure with your supervisor before making home visits. If there is an unusually large, contaminated dressing, another bag may be needed. The family should be taught how to discard all dirty equipment safely.
6. When the visit is completed, clean the used equipment and wash your hands before replacing equipment in the bag. Never reenter the bag unless you have washed your hands.
7. Close the bag and leave it in a clean area until you are ready to leave.

REMEMBER

- The contents of the bag are considered clean. When items from the bag are used, they must be cleaned before they are put back in the bag (see section on universal blood and body fluid precautions).
- The floor is considered a dirty area—never put your bag on the floor.
- Newspaper is considered clean and can be used if other items, such as bags, are unavailable.
- Place handwashing supplies—soap and paper towels—at the top of the bag where they can be easily reached.
- When not in use, the bag should be kept latched. Keep the bag out of sight when traveling in the car. Bring the bag in at the end of the day since extremes in temperature can damage equipment.
- Avoid bringing the bag into particularly dirty homes or where a client has a communicable disease. Prepare a small bag with the specific equipment you will need. Include in that bag, another bag in which to put back your cleaned equipment.
- Use the client's equipment as much as possible.

As mentioned, you will begin the intervention part of the visit by using the soap in the nursing bag and washing your hands. Always wash your hands before starting the visit. Following the handwashing procedure, the implementation of the care plan begins with such activities as teaching, direct care (e.g., a wound dressing), or assessment of the client's physiological or psychosocial status. While coordinating these activities, the home care nurse is constantly observing the client, the family, and the environment to determine if some modifications need to be made in the plan of care. It is important that the home care nurse involve the client and family or the significant other at every step of the implementation process. If the primary purpose of the visit is for the home care nurse to perform a dressing change, the nurse can be describing the procedure or the wound as the care is being performed. This will help the client and family to feel like active participants in the care. Once the implementation of the care plan is complete, the nurse should gather any equipment used and wash her hands. If equipment, such as thermometers, need to be washed or disposed of, it can be done at this time also.

In closing the visit, you will want to review the care the client is assuming or any aspects of the care plan that are particularly confusing. You will also set up an appointment for the next home visit and remind the client that he will receive a telephone call on the day of the visit to confirm the appointment. Although clients may devise their own system of remembering when visits are scheduled, if a client is having a particularly difficult time remembering when the home care nurse will come, marking a large calendar with the visit days is often useful.

The Post-Visit Stage. The home visit is not complete at the time you leave the client's home. Many activities comprise the post-visit stage and need to be done before your responsibilities are fulfilled. Based on the data collected during the home visit, revisions of the care plan may be indicated. You may have identified a new problem that should be added to the problem list and documented in the record, or resolved a problem that should be noted as such. Revision of any and all aspects of the care plan is completed following the home visit.

One of the most significant activities in the post-visit stage is the documentation of the interaction. Not only does documentation allow for communication between nurses and other health care providers, it provides the basis for reimbursement. There are many ways that documentation is accomplished, and you need to be thoroughly familiar with the system used by your agency. Refer to the section on home care documentation in Chapter 3.

An important post-visit activity is the communication of important information to other health care providers working with the client. It is during this stage that you may need to call the primary care provider to report the client's current condition. Case conferences with other disciplines involved (e.g., physical therapy, occupational therapy, social worker, nutritionist) may occur during this stage. Intra-agency communication is also a necessary part of this stage. If another nurse is serving as primary care nurse for the client, a brief verbal report of the visit is indicated, but the documentation on the client's chart should outline what was done on the visit and the client's status. At times, a report to the nursing supervisor is also indicated.

Referral to community agencies is also a part of post-visit activities. For example, if you determine that a client needed Meals on Wheels, you may make the referral in the client's home or wait until returning to the agency. Remember, always ask permission to use the client's telephone and make only local calls. If there is a chance that the referral source will ask for information that should not be stated in front of the client or family, make the referral at the agency.

Finally, you must care for any equipment that is to be returned to the agency and replenish your nursing bag with equipment and supplies. An ample supply of soap, paper towels, aprons, and other disposable supplies should be in your bag at all times. Agency policy will identify specific items to be carried in your bag. It is most helpful to replenish the bag at the completion of the home visit rather than at the beginning of the next day since you will have a clear memory of what equipment was used that day.

The home visit is the single most important tool for a home care nurse. As a guest in the client's home, you must recognize how certain behaviors have an impact on the implementation of the client's care. There are three phases in the home visit process; pre-visit activities, visit activities, and post-visit activities. The effective use of the nursing bag involves a technique that is carried out in a logical way during every visit. If all the phases of the home visit process are carried out in order, you will become an efficient and effective practitioner of home care nursing.

TEST YOURSELF

1. Write your own definition of home care nursing.

2. How do home care standards relate to your practice?

3. Identify three differences between hospital and home care nursing.

4. List the six rules of developing meaningful and understandable goals.

5. Discuss how you feel about doing home visits.

6. On your first home visit, using Figure 2–4 as your guide, write down the activities you completed, and compare these with the activities listed in the book. Based on this evaluation, what would you do differently next time?

7. What are the infection control measures used by your agency?

8. You are going for a home visit to a patient with an extremely unclean house. What are the most important aspects of bag technique in this situation?

9. Mr. Powell is a 68-year-old man who has a 10-year history of emphysema. He retired 3 years ago from an upholstery company where he worked most of his adult life, and he lives with his wife and two cats in a three-room apartment on the second floor of a house. He has two grown sons who live in the area, one who works at the same upholstery company as he did. His wife does not work outside the home but spends her days doing volunteer work with her friends for the local church.

   Mr. Powell was recently discharged from the hospital following an acute respiratory infection. Prior to admission to the hospital, Mr. Powell was able to go up and down the stairs several times during the day and was fairly independent in his ADLs. Following this respiratory infection, Mr. Powell was discharged from the hospital in an extremely weakened state with oxygen, several medications, and orders to avoid stairs. He experiences shortness of breath after walking 10 feet, and this frightens him. He states, "I just don't know what to do when I get so short of breath." Home care nursing was ordered for respiratory assessment, medication teaching, and assessment of the home environment.

   Using the nursing care plan of your agency, develop a brief nursing care plan for the Powell family. After you have finished identifying the nursing diagnoses, write the goals, develop interventions, and identify ways to evaluate the interventions. Discuss the care plan with your supervisor.

Documentation and Quality Assurance in Home Care

OBJECTIVES

Upon completion of this chapter, the reader will be able to identify

1. Standards and principles of documentation common to all types of nursing practice
2. The purposes of the parts of the chart
3. The five criteria a client must meet to be eligible for home care services under Medicare
4. The critical elements in documentation on Medicare forms 485 and 486
5. The aspects of a quality assurance program and the measures commonly used to evaluate each aspect
6. The significance of the interrelationship between structure, process, and outcome

KEY CONCEPTS

- **Standards and guidelines of documentation**

- **Five basic criteria for Medicare coverage**

- **How to complete forms 485, 486, and 487**

- **Documenting to satisfy Medicare regulations**

- **Structure–Process–Outcome aspects of quality assurance**

AGENCY-SPECIFIC MATERIAL NEEDED

- Forms 485, 486, and 487
- MIS manual
- Agency clinical record
- HIM–11 manual and agency supportive material
- NAHC videotape on documenting on forms 485, 486, and 487

- Procedure for certification and recertification
- Agency mission or philosophy
- Agency objectives
- Outcome measure instrument
- Organizational chart
- New staff nurse's job description

INTRODUCTION

Documenting the care given to a home care client is just as important as the quality of care provided. The chart review of clients used to assure that the care given meets clinical standards is an important aspect of an agency's quality assurance program. Third party payors use the client record also to justify payment for all home health services, including paraprofessionals. In this chapter the subjects of documentation and quality assurance in home care are combined, first, because they represent essential components of home care nursing practice, and second, because there are many differences between documentation and quality assurance practices in home care and in an institutional setting. In these two critical areas, the home care nurse must be both concerned about documenting care regarding reimbursement and involved in quality assurance issues in all of the agency's services. This chapter also goes into detail about the specific regulations for documenting care for Medicare clients and includes a discussion of legal considerations to help the nurse understand why implementing appropriate documentation techniques are essential for safe home care nursing practice.

DOCUMENTATION

Content, Practice, and Procedures

The home health care record is a written account of the client's history, status, and progress and usually contains a physician's plan of treatment (doctor's orders), client care forms, and business and financial data. It is the data base for planning individualized care for the client and serves to communicate information to all health professionals involved in the client's care. It also serves an important legal function; it documents evidence for the client's worker's compensation, insurance, or litigation-related claims. It is, therefore, paramount that the home health nurse recognize the importance of quality documentation and value it as much as hands-on care for clients.

Not only is proper documentation necessary to justify reimbursement for third party payors, it is also the key to the nurse's and agency's protection from liability. The phrase "if it wasn't charted, it wasn't done" reminds us that the best evidence of an event is usually what is in writing, and since most malpractice claims occur long after the events take place, when recollection can be unclear, the written record is given great weight. The written record can be the best indicator of what actually happened since it was written at the time of the event(s).

Using the following guidelines will help to ensure that the home care nurse will meet practice standards required by the legal duty to communicate.

1. **The record must be accurate in all respects.** Poor documentation can lead to errors in the care of the client. For example, doctor's orders must always be up-to-date. Persons who care for the client on weekends or intermittent caregivers, such as student nurses, must be able to rely on the accuracy of orders for medication and treatment.

2. **The actual content of the record should contain measurable and objective information rather than subjective statements.** A statement made by a client can be recorded in quotation marks to indicate the source of the data. In general, conclusions should be avoided, and the actual data recorded. For example, instead of recording that a client is "not eating enough" (conclusion), measurable objective data, such as amount of weight loss, daily intake, or statements from family members should be noted. Such phrases as "client appears comfortable" are not helpful since no observations are recorded to support this conclusion.

3. **Initial and ongoing assessments and nursing interventions must be documented in the record.** The nurse should record who was notified of changes in the client's status, including times and dates, and any other follow-up care. There is a clear legal duty to communicate essential findings to those who need to know (e.g., the client's physician).

In a suit that involved documentation in the recovery room, the plaintiff won his case, in part, because of inadequate recording on his chart. (**Wagner vs. Kaiser Foundation Hospitals,** 1979). After surgery to correct a tear duct obstruction, the patient eventually sustained neurological damage as a result of the anesthesia and a period of subsequent hypoxia after surgery. During the approximately 2 hours he was in the recovery room, the nurses' notes showed the recording of his blood pressure and pulse at 15-minute intervals, but with no record of his respirations. The written nursing note entries stated the patient was "doing well" and that there were "no apparent complications." The defendant nurses stated that it was standard policy to observe and count respirations and that the information was not charted unless there was something unusual. The court concluded, however, that failure to monitor the patient's respirations properly led to his problem not being discovered. Since the respirations were not recorded, the jury was allowed to conclude that they were not assessed. Thus, even routine nursing care should be recorded, and one should not rely on the claim that "we always do it." This type of evidence would not be persuasive to a court.

In another malpractice case against a hospital for negligent treatment, the plaintiff presented evidence of failure to document as an indication that observations of circulation to his toes were not made (**Collins v. Westlake,** 1974). There was a written doctor's order to "watch condition of toes," even though the doctor testified that it was usually routine in such injuries for the nurses to check the circulation in the foot. The nurse who was on duty part of the evening stated that normally a nurse does not chart each observation every time the patient is checked and that usually only abnormal findings are recorded.

The only entries on the nurse's notes the night in question were as follows:

12:30 Unable to sleep. Milk given.
1:30 Awake—med for pain.
6:00 A good night—states he feels better. Left foot is cold—color is dusky—appears to have no feeling on foot. Dr. Hubbard notified. (**Collins v. Westlake,** 1974, p. 617).

On appeal, the court concluded that there was no evidence in the record of the case that the circulation in the plaintiff's foot was observed by the nurse on duty at any time between 11:00 PM and 6:00 AM on the days in question. Therefore, the nurse's failure to recognize the condition led to the dangerous impairment of circulation that resulted in the amputation of the patient's foot.

4. **In the home care situation it is important not only to document direct observations, but to indicate what was taught to family members and the client in order to ensure proper monitoring of his condition.** Client education documentation, including instruction to family members, needs to be an ongoing part of the record. In some cases, written instructions provided to the client and his family can be persuasive evidence that such instructions were given. In an emergency room case involving a claim by a mother that she was not instructed to observe her son for complications of a head injury after he was discharged, one of the issues was verbal versus written instructions (**Crawford v. Earl Long Memorial Hospital,** 1983). A dispute arose between the nurse who testified that she gave these instructions verbally and the mother of the plaintiff. If the instructions had been in writing, it would have helped substantiate the claim that the client received the information. Written instructions should not replace verbal explanations and discussion, however, but should be used as a supplement to them. It is also recommended that the nurse document evaluative statements re-

lated to the client's understanding of the instruction. For example, "Client correctly drew up 40 U of NPH insulin and administered it in left thigh". In cases when detailed or complex instructions are needed, standard written instructions should be given. These instructions should be reviewed and updated periodically by home care nurses and administrators at the agency. An example might be written instructions for tracheostomy care in the home.

In order to improve documentation of side effects from medications, one home health agency devised a system of peel-off medication labels for each drug to be placed in the client's record (Plastaras, 1987). On the client's drug profile sheet was listed each drug with a corresponding preprinted label listing side effects. By having the information in a quick and usable form, documentation was easier and the nurses could instruct clients more efficiently. This system is an example of an improved way to recognize complications of drug therapy and drug interactions. This system also helps the nurse and the agency protect themselves against potential liability in this area.

Basic Principles of Effective Documentation

It is important to keep in mind some of the basic principles of good documentation, including how to correct errors and ensure proper timing of entries. Errors should remain legible by drawing a single line through the incorrect material and initialing above the error. If a large amount of information is charted on the wrong record, a line should appear through it, with the statement "charted in error," or "charted on wrong record." One should *not* use correction fluid or erase on the chart. In no case should records be destroyed or substituted at a later date. Doing so can give the impression that there was an error made or that there was an attempt to cover up for a mistake. In a Connecticut case, a large verdict was entered in the plaintiff's favor after a finding of negligence on the part of the hospital staff, (**Pisel v. Stamford Hospital,** 1980). Part of the evidence presented at trial was that the director of nursing had ordered the staff to destroy the original notes and to rewrite the nursing notes surrounding the incident of the patient's injury. In upholding the lower court's judgment, the appeals court stated that the falsified record could be considered evidence of the hospital's awareness of its negligence.

Entries must also be made in a timely manner, since other caregivers may need to rely on the information, and the clinical record is the major means of communicating client data. If one remembers additional data not recorded at the time of a previous note, it should be included later as an addendum.

The nurse should avoid contradictions or inconsistencies in the chart and make sure that reports for scheduled tests are included. These reports should be stamped or initialed with the date and time received so there is no question as to when they became a part of the record. Likewise, negative or derogatory comments about clients or other providers should not be made. Proxy charting, or signing for care given by someone else, is not a good practice. Countersigning, for example an RN signing with a home health aide, would be proper if the RN is responsible for the case through proper delegation of tasks to the other caregiver. It should be clear who actually delivered the care.

Other charting pointers include not using nonstandard abbreviations, since they could be misinterpreted. All phone conversations with the client, physician, or home care providers should be documented in the record. Any instructions to the client to make an appointment or follow-up with his physician should be noted. The client's failure to keep appointments with the home care nurse or others can provide evidence of the client's failure to comply with the recommended plan of treatment. This could later be used to help the agency establish the client's contributory negligence for an alleged injury and in some states could negate his claim or reduce the liability of others.

Documentation of Sensitive Areas of Practice

Questions arise as to what should be documented in situations that involve potentially sensitive areas of practice. One example might include when the nurse questions whether care by another health professional is inappropriate or substandard. Both case law and professional standards impose a duty on the nurse to report questionable care and, in some instances, to take further action beyond documentation to protect the client from harm.

The **American Nurses' Association (ANA) Code for Nurses With Interpretive Statements**, (1985) offers suggestions about how to handle questionable practice by another member of the health team. The first approach would be for the nurse to discuss the concern, and the possible harm it may cause to the client, with the person carrying out the questionable practice. If this doesn't yield any positive results, the findings should be reported to the appropriate authority within the agency or institution, following established formal channels. Every agency or practice setting should have a process for handling concerns of this type without fear of reprisal on the part of any employee who makes such a complaint. Written documentation of dates, times, observations, and events

that validate the nurse's concerns should be recorded. In some cases part of the documentation could be in a client's record, such as failure of a physician to return calls made on certain dates. Once there is legitimate concern raised, or a detrimental pattern established on the part of another caregiver, separate documentation should be completed in the form of incident reports or a log. All documentation should indicate clearly who was notified and what action, if any, was taken. This information should then be shared with the immediate supervisor who needs to have notice of any serious or immediate threat to the health care of the client.

If the problem is not corrected within the employment setting and continues to jeopardize the client's welfare and safety, other authorities may need to be contacted. An example would be a practice committee or state licensing board for specific categories of health care workers or professionals.

Some nurses think, mistakenly, that if they document substandard or questionable care in the client's record, that alone will meet the duty owed to the client. In fact, when nurses knew or should have known that medical care was substandard, courts have imposed a duty upon them to act beyond mere documentation. This point is illustrated by the case of **Utter v. United Hospital Center** (1977), a successful malpractice case against both a hospital and physician. The patient presented persuasive evidence that the nurses did not take proper steps to ensure his safety. Three days after the plaintiff had a cast put on in the emergency room, he showed signs of deteriorating. The nurses noted some of the abnormal findings in the record, but not others. The charge nurse testified that she called the physician and informed him of the patient's symptoms, but he did nothing further. A hospital policy manual stated that in such cases the supervisor and department chairperson should request consultation. Even if the data were properly documented in the patient's record, the court stated the nurses had an obligation to use positive action even beyond documentation.

Thus, even if the agency does not have a policy regarding what to do in this situation, the nurse has an obligation to act in circumstances where harm is likely to come to a patient. The steps that the nurse takes to meet this obligation should be carefully and objectively documented in the client's record.

Another case illustrates that nurses' complaints and action taken by review committees will be supported when proper steps are taken. In **Scappatura v. Baptist Hospital** (1978), the chief of staff and a hospital temporarily suspended a physician's privileges, acting on information from nurses that the postoperative measures taken by the physician were "extreme, unusual, and perhaps unsafe." The nurses informed their supervisor of the situation. The supervisor initiated the steps for suspension through a written memorandum of the incident to the medical director. The court upheld the emergency suspension, pending a later thorough investigation even though a formal due process hearing was not held.

A more difficult situation arises when the questionable practice that may have a detrimental effect on the client is by someone in the client's home who is not licensed or employed by an agency. For example, a home care nurse may question the activities of a person employed by the client as a homemaker or helper. The nurse's responsibility to the client in this situation will depend on a number of factors. The same general steps should be followed as outlined previously, with some modification, depending on the circumstances. For example, the home care nurse would first need to determine that the concern stems from the potential detrimental effect to the client's health since this is the basis of the nurse–client relationship. Personal concerns of the client, such as how he or she chooses to spend money or leisure time, need to be separated from genuine health concerns.

While the nurse is not responsible for the quality of care provided by private employees of the client, she does have a duty to the client at least to inform him or her of the concern and the basis for it. A proper notation of this conversation should be made in the client's record. If the client is fully competent, he or she has a right to take or withhold any action desired. If, however, the situation affects the care plan or the quality of care provided by the agency, there should be a mutually satisfactory resolution of the problem. An example would be if the nurse is teaching the client a sterile technique dressing change, but the homemaker follows a nonsterile procedure when the nurse is not there. If the nurse notices this, she must act on the situation, since the agency is responsible for the 24-hour care of the client with regard to the specified plan of care.

A different course of action may be required if the client is not competent. The nurse should then inform the client's family of the concern and let them make any decisions in the client's best interest. If no family member is available, state or local protective agencies may need to be informed. In an emergency situation, police or local authorities should be contacted, especially if illegal or unethical conduct is suspected. An example would be if the nurse has grounds to suspect that someone is taking advantage of the client by unauthorized use of his money or possessions.

Documentation of Child Abuse.

Another sensitive area of documentation arises when the nurse suspects that a child abuse or neglect situation exists in the home. This situation is reportable by statute to child welfare offices, and civil or criminal liability can follow from nonreporting if further abuse or neglect occurs. Suspected child abuse or neglect presents a challenging situation, since documentation and testimony by the home care nurse will likely be part of the evidence if a formal complaint is filed against an individual (see guidelines for testifying as a witness, Chapter 6). The nurse's primary role as the helper of the family seems to be in direct opposition to her role as an investigator gathering data that could have a negative or punitive effect on an individual.

The welfare and safety of the child must be at the core of her actions, but at the same time she must provide support and guidance for the family.

Documentation must contain precise and ongoing evaluation of the home environment, family interaction, and physical and emotional status of the child. Vague terms such as "seems" and "appears" should not be used since they indicate uncertainty.

When assessing and documenting information related to the child, any abnormal findings, such as bruises or cuts, need to be precisely located and measured. Growth charts should be used, with the child's data recorded on them. Developmental data should be included using such standard measurement tools as the Denver Developmental Screening Test (DDST) (Frankenburg & Dodds, 1969). The nurse should obtain a diet history and compare this to daily food and caloric requirements for the child. Food supplies should be checked to see if appropriate types and amounts of foods are available in the home. Parent–child interaction can be documented by recording whether the child is comforted by the parent and the parent's response to situations requiring discipline or safety measures.

Home environment in general needs to be considered and documented in the record, and conditions (e.g., appropriate temperature, cleanliness, sanitation, presence or absence of water, play, and sleeping space) should be noted. Safety considerations like open stairways or access to hazardous substances should be noted. Physical condition of the living quarters is often considered in a decision to remove a child from his home.

A detailed family history will often help clarify other stresses in the environment and may reveal ways that the family relieves stress. Along with this the nurse should document teaching or resources provided to the family to cope with situational crises. It is also important to determine the parent's perception of his role as a parent and whether expectations for the child are developmentally appropriate. Abusive parents sometimes have unrealistic expectations for the child, expecting behavior appropriate for an older child.

The child's emotional health and environment may be difficult to assess and document. That assessment should be based on observations of parent–child interaction, presence of toys or other stimulation in the environment, and the child's overall behavior. Emotional abuse of the child, although difficult to prove, may be evidenced by extreme perfectionism by the parent or constant belittling of the child's efforts to perform tasks. Any such behavior should be objectively noted in the record.

Jane L. Helberg suggests that a community health nurse may be aided in balancing conflicting roles with the abusive family by contracting with them for mutually agreed upon services (Helberg, 1983). The nurse can list broad teaching goals relating to the child's developmental level and behavior, improving the coping behavior and responses of the parent, and assisting in advocacy for better conditions for the family related to housing and finances. The parents could agree to work with the nurse to help alter the conditions that initiate the abusive behavior. Any failure of the parents to keep appointments or refuse services should be documented, since this serves as important evidence in any subsequent court proceeding.

Documentation of Elder Abuse. Just as is the case with children, the home care nurse may become involved in a situation where an elderly person is being neglected or abused. Elder abuse is reportable in most states. The principles underlying documentation are the same whether the client is a child or an older individual. The nurse should check with her supervisor regarding the regulations and procedures in your state.

The Home Care Chart

Unlike the hospital chart, which includes such things as doctor's notes, laboratory data, and test reports in addition to the nurse's notes, the home care chart includes only notes from the involved home care disciplines. The amount of charting the nurse must do in homecare is usually more extensive than that required in a hospital setting. The home care chart is used by the agency to document client needs and services provided and to produce a tangible legal record of all activities performed by the agency for the client. Pieces of documentation from the chart may be submitted to third party payors, including Medicare, to justify payment for services provided.

The content of home care charts varies from agency to agency, and the specific information included in the record is dictated by agency policies and state and federal regulations. To assure compliance with the requirements, often specific forms are used so that information can be easily documented and efficiently reviewed. Standardized care plans, such as the one described in Chapter 2 and shown in Appendix 3, are used frequently in home care charts.

Preprinted **flow sheets** are also useful for recording such basic data as vital signs and intake and output so that ongoing information and changes can be easily evaluated and interventions planned. Flow sheets that use check marks, numbers, or short phrases to cut down on charting time are often used for various parts of the home care chart. An example of a flow sheet for a patient with coronary artery disease and myocardial infarction is found in Figure 3–1. If a flow sheet is used for a care plan it might include a listing of the specific subjective and objective data to be assessed, the teaching required, procedures to be performed, and related nursing goals. Information on flow sheets can refer the reader to a narrative section that would then explain the observation in greater detail.

Although there may be some variation in charts and forms, all home health agencies include the chart components listed in this chapter. As each component is discussed in this section, the new staff nurse should have a copy of the agency's record available so that she can refer to the components in the agency's record as they are discussed.

Intake Form. The intake form contains the initial client information received by the agency when the client is referred for service. This data is usually taken over the telephone by the person in the agency responsible for taking referral information. The form includes basic demographic information, a brief history of the client's illness and past problems, preliminary physician's orders, current medications, and specific services ordered.

Physical Data Base. This data base includes findings from the initial nursing assessment, the client's past medical problems, mobility, and safety concerns.

Psychosocial and Socioeconomic Data Base. This section includes information about the client's lifestyle before his current illness, available support systems, emotional factors related to the client's current problems, and concerns about adequacy of housing, food and other issues that affect the home care plan. It may be in this section that billing information is gathered, including source of payment(s) for home care services, client's income and expenses, and any other forms the agency might require for financial records. Often, agencies choose to include the financial information in another section of the record.

Goals: Symptoms of CAD will be minimized. Medications and diet will be understood. Knowledge of risk reduction and symptoms to report will be demonstrated.

		DATES OF VISITS			
SUBJECTIVE	CAD pain				
	a. Location				
	b. Severity and duration				
	c. Precipitating factors				
	d. Accompanying symptoms: palpitations, vertigo, SOB, nausea, sweating				
	e. Measures of relief—effectiveness of TNG activity tolerance-degree of DOE, ADL tolerance				
OBJECTIVE	BP—indicate ⓇR & Ⓛsit				
	stand				
	Apical/radial pulse				
	Rhythm of pulse				
	Respiratory rate				
	Lung auscultation RUL				
	RML				
	RLL				
	LUL				
	LLL				
	Pedal edema Ⓡ				
	Measure instep and just above malleolus Ⓛ				
	Pedal/popliteal pulses Ⓡ				
	Ⓛ				
	Cyanosis/pallor				
TEACHING	Diet				
	Medications				
	Risk factors and reduction				
	Pacing of activity				
	Symptoms to observe for and report				

Figure 3–1. Standard Flow Sheet. Coronary Artery Disease (CAD)—Myocardial Infarction

Medication Information Record. The medication information record includes all client medications, both over-the-counter and prescription drugs. This part of the record may also include space to outline the side effects and teaching guidelines relevant to specific medications.

Nursing Care Plan. This section details the client problem list and nursing interventions developed by the nurse in collaboration with the client, family, physician, and other members of the health team.

Some agencies combine the care plan with the Health Care Financing Administration (HCFA) form 485 for all patients. Form 485 will be discussed later in this chapter. Included in the nursing care plan section are the patient's long- and short-term goals, which are used in the evaluation portion of the care planning process as well as in the agency's quality assurance program.

Nurse's Notes or Narrative. The narrative section of the record is often a plain sheet of lined paper that is used for a more detailed explanation of a problem identified on one of the flow sheets. A nursing narrative needs to be as clear, concise, and brief as possible without losing meaningful content. It is important to document the nurse's direct observations and comments made by the client on the narrative but not to repeat the information already recorded on the flow sheet. Since the purpose of the flow sheet is to give a picture of the client and chronicle the changes in the client's situation, it is not necessary to add to the narrative during or after each home visit if no outstanding problems need clarification.

The narrative may be used as the specific place to pull together nursing observations and interventions to present a total picture of the client's condition. For instance, a client has congestive heart failure (CHF). On this visit the nurse observes pitting edema of the feet and rales that the base of the right lung which are negative changes based on flow sheet data from previous visits. The nurse would record clearly in the narrative the symptoms that indicate that the client may be going into CHF, that she plans to consult with the physician regarding medication or a diet order change, and the need for increased frequency of nursing visits to evaluate further the client's condition and response to any medication or diet changes. By using the narrative in this constructive way, the flow sheet will include the quantitative changes observed in the client (edema, rales), and on the narrative the nurse can document the subjective feelings of the client and her professional assessment, diagnosis, and plan. This use of the narrative results in a very efficient and effective way of documenting.

Physician's Orders. The physician's orders section of the record includes the specific medical orders for the client. In this section there may be a separate form outlining the physician's original orders, filled out when the client is referred or admitted to the service. Often, additional orders using the agency's form are sent after admission. During the client's relationship with the agency, orders are renewed and telephone orders for updates or changes are sent as needed. Parameters regarding renewal of physician's orders and procedures for verbal orders vary from agency to agency and often are guided by rules of various payment sources.

Physicians' orders include such information as diagnoses, medications, diet, allergies, prognoses, activity limitations, and specific home health services ordered (e.g., nursing, therapy, home health aide). The period of time covered by the orders should be spelled out on the form and, although the time period is usually based on agency policy, government regulation, or both, 2 months is common. If the client is newly discharged from a hospital or other institution,

that facility may send orders on a standardized form that is used state- or citywide. Once the client has been assessed in the home setting, if additional services or skills are needed, additional physician's orders outlining these must be sent after a telephone call is made to the doctor.

In home care, the nurse takes information from the intake sheet, data gathered at the initial visit, and the client and family's perception of need. The nurse then completes the physician's order form, which is then forwarded to the doctor for signature. The physician verifies the orders written on the form, adds any other information necessary, signs the form, and returns it to the agency's office.

Ideally, every agency should have a simple, separate physician's order form available for verbal physician orders, such as for a change in dressing procedure or medication. Some insurance companies may require certain statements or information in the physician's orders. For example, the words "medically necessary" might be needed in the orders if nurse's aide services are required. The nurse should check the client's individual policy requirements before writing the physician's orders; this is usually done in collaboration with the agency's billing department.

Medicare (a federal insurance plan) requires the use of a federally printed form—number 485—as the physician's order form. Many agencies have opted to use form 485 as the physician's order form for all clients. Medicare also uses a billing form—number 486—and provides a form—number 487—for additional information that won't fit on forms 485 or 486. The rules, regulations, and forms used in the Medicare program will be outlined in the next section.

Medicare

Medicare is a federal insurance program for many older or disabled people in the United States. It is important for the home care nurse to understand Medicare for two reasons

1. The nurse's judgment, based on her first home evaluation and review of the physician's orders, determines whether the client's services are reimbursable under Medicare.
2. The nurse's documentation is scrutinized by Medicare to determine whether the client's services are reimbursable by Medicare.

Medicare is governed by the Health Care Financing Administration (HCFA). HCFA contracts with insurance companies to process Medicare bills. The federal government has divided the country into ten regions with an insurance company in each region responsible for administering the Medicare home care benefit. These insurance companies are called fiscal intermediaries (FIs). The home health agency sends bills to the FIs on a monthly basis. Accompanying the bills are copies of the client's form 485 (physician's orders), form 486 (billing form and medical update), and form 487 (addendum), if needed.

The FI hires nurse reviewers who read forms 485, 486, and 487, and determine if the client and home care services meet the coverage criteria for the Medicare home care benefit. If documentation clearly indicates that the client's condition and the care provided meet the Medicare criteria for reimbursement, the bill is paid. If the FI does not find the documentation to be clear regarding their criteria for reimbursement, they will send a request for more information (form 488) to clarify the issue. This usually involves copying portions of the nursing record to provide the requested information.

It is important then, to

1. Understand the basic five criteria for Medicare coverage, so that the home care nurse can make an informed decision regarding reimbursement for care provided
2. Understand what should be included in nursing documentation to show clearly that reimbursement criteria have been met

The Five Basic Criteria for Medicare Coverage. The basic criteria for Medicare coverage are explained in detail in the Health Insurance Manual –11 (HIM-11), written by HCFA (Medicare, 1989). The agency should have a copy of this, and the nurse should read sections 203–206.7. The home health agency may have additional material that will help the nurse understand the manual. Some FIs have developed handbooks containing HIM-11 sections 203–206.7 that have additional, clarifying information regarding documentation and coverage issues. The National Association for Home Care (NAHC) has produced videotapes explaining these sections in detail. They may be available for study through the home health agency. A client must meet all *five* criteria to have services reimbursed by Medicare.

Reasonable and Necessary-HIM–11 Section 203.1–203.3. To be covered under Medicare, services must be "reasonable and necessary." The terms reasonable and necessary are not clearly defined by Medicare; the decision whether this criterion is met is based on "the patient's health status and medical needs as reflected in the home health plan of care and medical record." Intermediaries will assume the type and frequency of services ordered are reasonable and necessary unless objective clinical evidence clearly indicates otherwise or there is a lack of clinical evidence

to support coverage. A coverage determination may be made based on a review of HCFA forms 485, 486, and 487. The home care nurse must provide clear documentation regarding the client's progress or lack of progress, medical condition, functional losses, and goals.

Homebound—HIM–11 Section 204.1. A client must be considered essentially homebound to be eligible for home care benefits under Medicare. This means that the client leaves home only with some difficulty with mobility and only for medical appointments or a *rare* trip for something nonmedical, such as a haircut. A client who is very depressed or fearful and so for psychological reasons will not leave home is also considered homebound. The client is considered homebound if the absences from the home are infrequent or for periods of relatively short duration, or are attributable to the need to receive medical treatment. Homebound criteria may be met when the beneficiary attends adult day care when the purpose is related to the client receiving medical care.

Plan of Care—HIM–11 Section 204.2. The client's "plan of care must contain all pertinent diagnoses, including the beneficiary's mental status, types of services, supplies, and equipment ordered, the frequency of the visits to be made, prognosis, rehabilitation potential, functional limitations, activities permitted, nutritional requirements, medications and treatments, safety measures to protect against injury, discharge plans, and any additional items the home health agency or physician choose to include."

Skilled Services—HIM–11 Sections 204.4–205 The services rendered must be skilled, (ie, they must require the specialized skills of a trained nurse or physical or speech therapist). Medical social work (MSW) and home health aide (HHA) services are not considered skilled services and, therefore, will not be reimbursed by Medicare if they are the *only* services needed by a home care client. Medical social work and HHA are dependent services and can only be given if one or more of the other three skilled services are also needed. Reimbursement of occupational therapy (OT) is unlike the other disciplines mentioned. The nurse should read the agency's manual regarding OT. The determination of whether a service is skilled is made on the inherent complexity of the service, the condition of the client, and accepted standards of medical and nursing practice.

This section of the manual should be read very carefully, and the nurse should be familiar with the requirements for other skilled services, but must be completely comfortable with the criteria for skilled nursing service. Skilled nursing services encompass three major areas: **skilled observation and assessment,** such as determining signs of CHF; **teaching,** such as instructing a client about new medications (the side effects and effect on the client's condition); and **performing skilled procedures,** such as intravenous (IV) therapy or wound packing with a sterile dressing. The HIM–11 manual goes into detail with numerous examples. The nurse should ask her supervisor any questions that she may have.

Criteria for home health aides is found in section 206.2. Since the home care nurse will be determining the need for home health aides and supervising their care, she will also need to be familiar with this section of the manual.

Intermittent-Part-time—HIM-11 Sections 205.1C and 206.7. Medicare specifies that home care services must be provided on an intermittent basis. This means that under normal circumstances, home visits by any discipline will not be made daily. The HIM-11 (section 205.1.C) indicates Medicare will pay for skilled nursing care 7 days a week for a short period of time which Medicare sees as 2 to 3 weeks. Daily visits, for example, might be needed to teach a family member to do a sterile dressing involving packing of the wound. There may also be a few cases involving unusual circumstances where the patient's prognosis indicates the medical need for daily skilled services will extend beyond 3 weeks. As soon as the patient's physician makes this judgment, which usually should be made before the end of the 3 week period, the home health agency must forward medical documentation justifying the need for such additional services and include an estimate of how much longer daily skilled services will be required.

Skilled nursing and aide services can be provided on what Medicare calls a part-time basis or up to a maximum of 35 hours per week of up to 8 hours combined time each day. Such coverage would, however, need to be determined on a case by case basis. Section 206.7 of the HIM-11 Manual defines part-time as any number of days per week:

• Up to and including 28 hours per week of skilled nursing and home health aide services combined for less than 8 hours per day; or

• Up to 35 hours per week of skilled nursing and home health aide services combined for less than 8 hours per day subject to review by fiscal intermediaries on a case by case basis, based upon documentation justifying the need for and reasonableness of such additional care.

Documentation for Medicare. The home care nurse's documentation on forms 485, 486, and 487 is submitted to the FI for medical review. Information on these forms must be supported by information in the cli-

ent's clinical chart. It is important that the home care nurse understand how to document not only on the forms 485, 486, and 487 but in the clinical record as well, which was covered in an earlier section in this chapter.

Documentation on Forms 485, 486, and 487. The HCFA forms 485, 486, and 487 consist of many boxes that require specific information. Each of these boxes with its corresponding number is called a *locator.* The HCFA has produced a workbook and videotape that describe in detail, locator by locator, how to fill out forms 485, 486, and 487. These tools can be helpful. If the home health agency does not have these available, the nurse can check any written guidelines developed by the agency to guide her through the completion of these forms.

Form 485. Form 485 is the signed physician's order form. For Medicare purposes it encompasses home health certification and plan of treatment and

1. Is the plan of treatment for the attending physician only
2. Requires the attending physician's signature
3. Is reviewed at least every 60 days
4. Is totally prospective
5. Is completed with each certification and recertification
6. Includes Medicare covered and non-Medicare covered services
7. Can have no locator left blank

The following sections outline suggestions on how to complete some of the more important locators. It will be helpful to have copies of forms 485, 486, and 487 available for reference during this section. When the new staff nurse has completed the reading, the nurse's observations should be validated with the supervisor. The supervisor may have additional hints to make the understanding of these forms easier.

Form 485—Sections 11, 12, and 13. In recording diagnoses and surgical procedures the nurse must be sure to include any that would help to justify the services being requested even if they are not directly related to the reason for the current services. For example, if a fractured hip is the principal diagnosis but the client also has multiple joint arthritis, osteoporosis, and chronic obstructive pulmonary disease (COPD), the nurse could be sure to include these under section 13. They indicate that the client has complicating factors and help to justify a longer duration and greater frequency of visits for physical therapy. If a newly insulin dependent diabetic client also is a bilateral amputee and has severe COPD, be sure to include these diagnoses as they help document homebound status.

Form 485—Sections 18, A and B, 19, and 20. As these sections are filled out, the nurse should think about the client's limitations. Record the lowest functioning level the patient exhibits. For example, avoid Section 18.B, 7 "independent at home" and Section 18.B–C "no restrictions" as they may trigger the intermediary reviewer to question homebound status. Instead use 18.B #3 "up as tolerated," which doesn't indicate the same high level of functioning. Anyone who is independent at home is certainly up as tolerated. If the client is essentially oriented but often forgetful and at times agitated, Check off #3 "forgetful" and #7 "agitated" (under #19, Mental Status). By completing this section in this manner, the nurse reveals the client's lower functioning level and, therefore, shows he is more in need of the services requested.

Don't hesitate to use the "other" boxes in this section. For example, if the client has cancer with frequent nausea and vomiting that could be considered a limiting factor under #18.A (Functional Limitation), check off the "other" box and write in "nausea and vomiting." Under 18.B (Activities Permitted) "non-weight-bearing status on one leg" could be written in below the "other" box for a leg fracture patient. With a CVA client who is emotionally labile, include this observation in the "other" category under #19, Mental Status.

Form 485–Section 21. As previously indicated, Medicare considers skilled care to be assessing, observing, teaching, and performing skilled procedures. The nurse should be sure to include the terms assessing, observing, and teaching in the doctor's orders in this section. This will help to avoid the use of words denoting minimal skill such as supervise, reinforce, or encourage. An example, using a client with a new colostomy who also had an exacerbation of her COPD and CHF postoperatively, would be

> Skilled nursing (SN) to assess cardiorespiratory status and response to new medications, bowel status, and skin integrity around stoma. Teach colostomy care, bowel regime to help normalize stool, and diet. Also teach correct medication use and the effects and side effects of meds, pacing of activity, COPD, CHF disease processes, and symptoms for the client to observe and report.

For the client with a coronary artery bypass graft (CABG), who developed arrthymias and cardiac arrest, and then urinary retention postoperatively, the nurse might write

> SN to assess cardiac status, particularly rate, rhythm, and response to new medications, healing of incisions, intake and output, and amount of residual urine. Teach the client medications and symptoms of wound complications to observe and report. Teach self-catheterization using clean technique and a #16 F. straight catheter.

When writing direct care skills in your orders be sure to note the specific procedure you will be performing. For example, the directions could be phrased as "SN to pack wound bid with a wet or dry saline dressing," or "SN to insert a #18 Foley catheter with 5 cc balloon 1 × mo × 2 mos and 4 × prn for Foley dysfunction."

In this section the amount, frequency, and duration of visits must be detailed. The key is to estimate the number of visits which will cover any unexpected visits—perhaps a new problem has developed or the client is learning more slowly than expected. It is essential to anticipate a few prn visits or estimate visit ranges to adjust for changes in the patient's condition. For example, for a CHF client with new medications, diet, and little understanding of the disease, the nurse might write this section in two ways:

- 1. "SN to visit 4×/wk × 1 wk, 2×/wk × 2 wks, 1×/wk × 2 wks, and prn × 3 if problems arise with client's condition or teaching progresses slowly." This approach allows for a 5-week parameter of coverage. If the client's condition warrants additional visits beyond those initially requested, a copy of form 486 in modified format can be completed and sent to the intermediary with the next billing along with a copy of the physician's order to cover the change. The box indicating "modified" must be checked in locator 12 on Form 486.p
- 2. "SN to visit 4–5×/1wk, 2–3×/4wks, 1–2×/4wks." This approach develops a 9-week parameter of care that will cover nursing visits until the next certification period (60 days). By doing this you will have orders for the entire certification period and not need to send additional, interim orders unless the visits needed go beyond those in the original order.

The home care nurse can discuss these two approaches with the supervisor and explore further the agency's policies in this matter.

Form 486. Form 486 encompasses the data needed by FIs to make coverage determinations on home health claims. Form 486

1. Reflects orders from all physicians contributing to the clients's plan of care
2. Is completed with each certification, recertification, as a modifier, or with denials
3. Includes Medicare-covered services only
4. Is completed at the time of billing for certification and recertification, or at the point of change for modifiers and denials

5. Can be either retrospective, prospective, or both, depending upon the time of completion
6. Includes physician's new orders
7. Can have no locator left blank

It can be difficult to determine when form 486 is to be completed and which dates of service should be included. It will be helpful for the home care nurse to remember the following:

- Locators 1–8, 11–15, and 17–21 should be filled out at the time form 485 is completed.
- Locators 9–10, 16, and 22 should be completed at the end of whichever month is entered in the date of the certification period in locator 3 on the form 486.

For **certification** (first time form 486 is completed), information will be included covering the period from the date of admission to the end of that same month. For recertification (subsequent copies of form 486), information included should cover 1) the reasons why home care needs to be extended into the next 60 day period, 2) an update of the clinical findings, and 3) projected amount of service needed in the next 60 day period. For example, the home care nurse should state the condition of the wound and any complications which have occurred that prevented healing as well as the modified plan for further treatment.

It is important to remember that this section contains the nurse's legal orders, so the form must be complete in its listing of all skills that the nurse will be performing and those for which a physician's order must be included. Form 486 must be filled out comprehensively, indicating all areas of assessment and teaching possible to indicate the need for skilled services. The general principles of this section apply to *all* skilled services requested.

Form 486—Section 16. This locator serves four purposes:

1. **New orders/treatments.** The home health agency is to record any new orders, treatments, or changes and associated date(s) from the time form HCFA–485 is completed to the time form HCFA–486 is completed. It must include all changes in physicians' orders reflecting changes in client status. It must also list updated information in chronological order. Note: Document only if needed.
2. **Clinical facts.** The home health agency should record significant clinical findings for each discipline, incorporating all symptoms and changes in the client's condition, including dates of visits made as circumstances required. Upon certification, enter clinical findings of the initial assess-

ment visit for all disciplines involved in the care plan. Describe the clinical facts about the client that require skilled home health services. Documentation should include specific dates.
3. **Summary from each discipline.** Document progress or nonprogress for each discipline.
4. **Optional space.** To expand from form HCFA–486, locator 10, "Date Last Contacted Physician" and locator 14, "Dates of Last Inpatient Stay." Note: Document in this section only as needed.

It is important in this section not to list just vital signs and other factual data but to literally tell a story in as concise a way as possible. This will persuade the intermediary beyond a doubt that the services requested are needed. It is important that negative data and problem areas be stressed. Chart teaching that needs to be accomplished and stress any knowledge deficits of the patient and family. The home care nurse must chart ways the client is at high risk for problems to develop and include relevant information from the client's hospital stay indicating complications or other problems that developed. Note the following examples of clinical data that could be included in this section. Both discuss the same client, but which really justifies the services requested?

The client has just been discharged from an acute hospital with a below the knee amputation of the right leg.

Example 1

SN: Right stump, incision had 3 × 1 cm separation on admission with serous, pink drainage saturating 2 4×4s. Now wound size 1 × 0.5 cm. Redness has decreased, serous drainage only. Able to ambulate well. Having difficulty breathing. Taking pain medication as required.

Example 2

SN: Wife has learned correct dressing change technique. Occasional cough, bi-basilar rales. LLE 2+ edema. Exertional dyspnea. Blood glucose 100. On admission, required pain medication q 4 hr. By 03/31/89, required medication only upon awakening and again at bedtime. Wound on right stump had 3 × 1 cm separation on admission with serous, pink drainage saturating 2 4×4s. Now wound size 1 × 0.5 cm., redness has decreased, serous drainage only.

PT: 20° flexion contracture right knee. Improved to 10° by 03/31/89. Required assist of one to transfer on admission and able to ambulate 30 feet. Now able to ambulate 50 feet with standby assist but requires assist of one to transfer. On 03/30/89, increased repetitions of theraband exercises to right hip flexors and extensors. As of 03/31/89, strength in right hip and quads remains F+. Cannot navigate stairs, inclines, or unlevel surfaces or get from floor to chair unassisted.

AIDE: Continues to require standby assist to ambulate. Requires assist to transfer. Has progressed from needing complete assistance with bathing to requiring assist only on his back, left lower extremity, and hair shampoo.

The second example certainly gives the reviewer clear reasons why assessing, observing, and teaching skills are needed and would justify increased visit frequency, at least initially.

Form 486—Section 17. This section expands on the check list on functional limitations of form 485. As in all documentation on forms 485, 486, and 487, the nurse must be sure that the client's chart will substantiate anything written. In completing the forms, the nurse must remember that functional limitations are not only such physical limitations as ambulation difficulties or activities of daily living (ADLs), but include such things as slowness to grasp new concepts, illiteracy, visual limitations, and anxiety.

To help establish homebound status, the nurse must be specific regarding physical or psychological limitations such as "client can only walk 20 feet before becoming severely dyspneic" or "client refuses to use stairs for fear of falling." In describing prior functional status, the greater the gap between abilities before the client became ill and the present, the better. This is especially true for PT requests. Most clients are weak following major abdominal surgery for cancer with creation of a colostomy. If the client was totally independent, however, and drove and played golf before surgery and now requires the assistance of one person to transfer or ambulate with a walker, then PT should be justified for strengthening and progressive ambulation.

Form 486—Section 19. In filling out this section, information about the actual environment should be included, for example, indicating the lack of durable equipment needed for care or a noisy home including five small grandchildren. The client's wife might be very anxious about her husband's condition and, thus, very slow to learn his care. These areas are important and exemplify the family/community focus of home care nursing.

Form 486—Sections 20 and 21. The Medicare requirement for clients to be homebound is partially determined by the answers to Sections 20 and 21. The answer to item 20 should be none in cases where the patient is homebound. Remember, "essentially homebound" status is needed by Medicare. Section 21 should indicate the client leaves only for periodical medical appointments. If the client is, upon occasion, not found at home by the home care nurse or regularly leaves for social purposes, he or she doesn't qualify for Medicare.

By reading this section on Medicare and the paperwork required by the nurse for reimbursable visits, it is understandable why some agencies do not choose to accept Medicare clients. Learning the criteria for Medicare and effectively filling in forms 485, 486, and 487 is time consuming and, therefore, costly. The handling of form 488, which asks for additional information for the fiscal intermediary's review, is also expensive, in terms of time, and additional time is spent appealing denials and keeping track of changes in the regulations and interpretations. Dealing with Medicare and the FIs can be frustrating when coverage for a client that was thought to be qualified is denied or when HCFA changes a procedure or a way of interpreting a set of criteria. Significant frustration can also be felt by both the client and family members. When the home care nurse understands the criteria, she can explain to the client certain aspects of the Medicare requirements and limitations.

Documentation for Medicare should use language found in the HIM–11 manual under the criteria for skilled services. This holds true for documentation on forms 485, 486, and 487 as well. Although the following guidelines are essential for Medicare clients, they also address sound clinical practice, are descriptive, and, therefore, can be used for all clients to document clearly the skilled level of care provided.

Documentation Hints

- Use words such as
  - Observation/assessment
  - Management/evaluation
  - Teaching/instruction
  - Performance of skilled procedures
- Documentation should support the reasonable potential for complications or ineffective healing
- Documentation must support the client's inability to perform a procedure (such as administer insulin) and the nonavailability of an able or willing caregiver. When there is a caregiver in the home, the documentation must indicate that the caregiver is unable or unwilling to perform specific procedures.
- When the teaching constitutes reinforcement, documentation should indicate any modifications or reinforcement needed in the home environment, for safety or effectiveness
- Document that the skills of a nurse are required based on
  - Inherent complexity of the service
  - Condition of the patient
  - Accepted standards of practice
- Key documentation questions
  1. Can the services be furnished safely and effectively without the skills of a nurse?
  2. Is the care consistent with the client's medical condition and accepted standards of practice?

- Document briefly the factors resulting in a high likelihood of complication or factors ensuring that essential skilled services are achieving the purpose to promote the client's recovery and safety
- Skilled management and evaluation involve a finding that recovery or safety can not be assured unless the total care, skilled or not, is planned and managed by a registered nurse
- Skilled management and evaluation require a specific physician's order when it is the only skilled service rendered. Check with your supervisor regarding regulations in Section 2.14.11 of The HIM 11 Manual.
- Document the reasons that the client's condition could change, leading to a subsequent acute episode or medical complication
- Document why skilled observation and assessment are needed to determine if treatment should be changed
- Coverage for a minimum of 3 weeks will be granted when documentation indicates a reasonable potential for medical complications or development of a further acute episode
- Always document any modifications made to the treatment or any additional medical procedures initiated as a result of nurse's assessments
- When documenting wound care, be specific regarding
  - Nature of drainage
  - Amount of drainage
  - Procedure performed
  - Amount and type of irrigation solution
  - Any edema, pain, or heat
  - Length and width of packing
  - Number and size of dressing(s) applied
  - Condition of surrounding area
  - Name of any topical ointments, creams, or other medications applied
  - Measurement and description of wound dimensions
- When documenting other skilled procedures, follow the same principles as in wound care. *Be specific and use details*
- Document facts, not opinions. Be objective, not subjective
- Documentation should be complete, accurate, and reflect the care actually given at each visit
- Documentation should be as brief and concise as possible
- Document the clinical findings. Indicate that the client remains unstable and needs further care, not that the client is improving. For example, a statement might read, "client's wound measures 3" long, ½" wide, and 1" deep. Last week it was 3½" long, ½" wide, and 1¼" deep," instead of "wound healing nicely"

- Each note should contain
  - Why the visit is necessary
  - Specific observations to substantiate why the visit is necessary
  - Skilled care given
- Care documented should relate to the client's diagnosis
- Use quantifiable, measurable, terms. Be technical, mathematical, and scientific
- When teaching, document client's and family's progress or lack of progress toward the goal. Elaborate on factors affecting the lack of progress

Continuity of Care

Continuity of care can involve seeing that optimal care is given on a 24-hour basis within one agency, or that optimal care continues if the client is transferred to another agency.

Aside from the client's chart, verbal reporting among professionals is very important. Conferences between professionals should be concise, stress the individual needs of the client, and indicate any special considerations for care. Such reporting should give the other professional a clear picture of what needs to be done for the client and how the care must be individualized so that the next professional has direction in providing the care. Clients can become very frustrated when they deal with a variety of caregivers, each of whom treats him or her differently or is confused about procedures and the plan of treatment.

In a home care agency the chart may not be readily available at times other than regular office hours. For very ill clients, who may call when the office is closed, an abbreviated chart containing information on diagnoses, care needed, and support systems for the client should be given to the "on call" nurse so she can handle any phone call or make a home visit with some knowledge of the client and care plan. For scheduled visits after regular office hours, an abbreviated chart, which includes flow sheets with procedures and descriptions of objective data, can be left in the home. Nurses could chart on the homebased record as well as the office chart. Agency policy dictates if this home-based record is an official part of the record or a worksheet used for communication among disciplines; in either case, a specific policy should outline how this written information is to be handled.

If a client is being seen by two home health agencies for different services, it is essential that the personnel from both agencies communicate and decide which will be the primary agency. This situation often happens if one agency is engaged for nursing and physical therapy and another agency provides the home health aide. The primary agency is usually responsible for the written orders and the supervision of the care given in the client's home. Certain states have regulations guiding such relationships between agencies.

If the client or family contracts with individuals such as a homemaker to care for the client at various times while a home health agency is caring for the client, the agency must determine the relationship they are to have with the individuals employed by the client. Each agency should have a policy governing the role that the nurse is to play in this situation and how the nurse shall interact with these persons. In this situation, it is essential that the family and client understand completely that they have the primary responsibility for the work performed by those persons.

If the care of a client is being transferred to another agency, written and verbal communication is needed. The new agency needs to know such things as the patient's diagnoses, the care that has been given, what future goals are identified, and specific orders, such as diet, treatments, and medications.

Discharging the Client. Planning for discharge from home care should begin during the first home visit. The nurse and client should plan the care that is needed and determine how and over what period of time this care can be accomplished. The section on contracting in Chapter 4 outlines this process completely. The nurse should help the client to understand what services can realistically be offered in the home setting and with what degree of frequency. The nurse, the client, and the client's family need to set goals together. Updating these goals periodically allows everyone involved to see clearly how objectives are being accomplished and when discharge can be anticipated.

Discharge from the home care agency services is often just as stressful for clients as is discharge from the security of a hospital. In most cases, discharge means the client has progressed to self- or family care and no longer requires the services of a professional nurse. At the time of discharge, families must have sufficient knowledge to cope with the day-to-day issues that arise in the client's care. They also need to know how to reach help in case of an emergency. The preparations the home care nurse makes for the discharge of the client must be clearly documented in the patient's record. The standard criteria for discharging a client from home care are

1. The goals for the client set out in the contract have been achieved.
2. The care (nursing, physical, or speech therapy) required by the client no longer is skilled.

3. The client is hospitalized and time of return to the home is unknown.
4. The client refuses further service by the agency.
5. The client moved or is moving out of the agency's service area.
6. The service now needed for the client is not available from the home health agency.
7. There is no funding available in the agency to provide the care, so client is referred elsewhere.
8. The client died.
9. The home situation is unsafe, and intermittent care is not adequate to meet the client's needs. In this situation, agency policies should be consulted to address the issues of abandonment.

Although all of these situations are applicable for discharge, there are times when a client wants to continue receiving home services on a private pay basis. In this case, the nurse should consult the agency's policy manual or a supervisor (Humphrey, 1986).

Recording the discharge in the client's record simply involves clearly stating the reason for discharge and indicating how the goals were achieved. A verbal or written summary of care given, the status of the client at discharge, and the reason for discharge is the minimum of information that should be communicated to the client's physician. Individual agencies may have additional information or a form that outlines the data that is to be sent to the physician.

When a client is discharged from home care services to another agency, (e.g., an extended care facility) the home care nurse can serve to ease the transition between home and nursing home by informing the staff of the way in which the client accomplished ADLs at home. Whatever information the nurse can provide to ease the transition should be communicated to the other agency personnel orally and in writing. This is often done using an interagency communication form.

QUALITY ASSURANCE IN HOME CARE

Overview

Nurses have always been concerned about the quality of care their clients received. Implementation of measures that evaluate the quality of care have received more attention and become more organized since the mid sixties. Federal legislation, coupled with the increasing consumer rights movement in the United States, has fueled the development of rigorous quality assurance programs in home care agencies and promises even more emphasis on quality assurance in the future. Most important, the recognition by the nursing profession of its responsibility to evaluate itself has resulted in the implementation of quality assurance programs that monitor the care that clients receive. A quality assurance program is a comprehensive agencywide system that measures the quality of care provided by identifying those factors that affect the quality of care.

One of two questions that need to be addressed when discussing quality assurance is, **What** is being assured? Quality assurance involves the accountability of the provider delivering care to clients and measuring the quality of that care. Quality assurance also involves the governing of nursing practice so that all clients will receive care that is equal to or better than the standard of care for clients who have like characteristics. Standards of care are comprehensive guidelines that define the ideal nursing interventions or behaviors to be performed in specific situations. This means simply that if the home care nurse is caring for a client with a specific illness, there are certain required interventions to be performed. For example, if the nurse is caring for a client with a myocardial infarction (MI) and the standards of care for clients with an MI minimally include assessment of the peripheral vascular status, the client's peripheral vascular status must be assessed on each visit. Sources for the standards of care include nursing textbooks, journal articles, the American Nurse's Association, and precedent established through judgments in court cases. So, the answer to the question of what is being assured, is: high-quality care, which meets or exceeds set standards that will lead to accountability by professionals to consumers of that care.

The second question is, **To whom** is the nurse accountable? The nurse is primarily accountable to the client for the quality of care that is provided. The client has the right to expect the highest quality of care available within the constraints of applicable rules and regulations. The delivery of home care is client specific, and as such, the client should play as active a role as possible in the delivery of that care. As the recipient of care, the client pays the greatest price for inadequate or inferior care, not only in dollars, but also in risk to health.

In addition to the nurse's accountability to the client, the nurse is also accountable to the employing agency, which expects a certain degree of excellence in professional practice and to the third party payors, who pay for the services that are performed and who expect a professional level of treatment in exchange for the expense of a registered nurse. Since the advent of Medicare, home health agencies have been required to monitor the quality of care to clients in various ways in order to attain and maintain status as Medicare certified agencies. Other third party payors,

such as private insurers, have also required the implementation of quality assurance programs for home health agencies.

A fourth category of accountability is the nurse's professional peer group, which demands that high-quality care be provided. Although the home care nurse is independent in practice, peer relationships are an important element in professional growth and job satisfaction. Peers can be helpful in discussing a difficult or challenging client situation and in providing emotional support. As a member of a professional group, the nurse must also be willing to provide emotional support and professional consultation to her colleagues.

The nurse's responsibility for the quality of care provided to clients is described in the figure, Standards of Home Care Practice in chapter 2. As discussed in chapter 2 the standards of practice were developed by the American Nurses' Association as a guide to the practice of home care. The seventh of those standards states, "The nurse participates in peer review and other means of evaluation to ensure quality of nursing practice. The nurse assumes the responsibility for professional development and contributes to the professional growth of others."

To summarize, the concept of quality assurance is not new to the nursing profession. Nurses have always been concerned about the quality of care their clients receive but have not always known how to measure it. Since 1965, federal legislation and an increase in consumer activism in the United States have fueled the development and growth of quality assurance programs in home care nursing, and those programs can reveal specific, measurable data concerning the quality of care provided. The home care nurse is accountable to the client, her employer, third party payors, and nursing peers. Because of the extent of her accountability, it is imperative that the home care nurse understand all areas of quality assurance.

Quality Assurance Program

A quality assurance program is a comprehensive system that measures the quality of care provided throughout the agency as viewed from several perspectives. An integral part of any quality assurance program is the implementation of measures that will improve the quality of care provided. In order to measure the quality of care a client receives, three areas have traditionally been assessed; structure, process, and outcome (Barlow, 1989). The interrelationship of these three components forms the essence of any quality assurance program. Any of these elements studied individually cannot provide the evaluator and the agency with the necessary data on which to base decisions regarding the quality of care that clients receive. The three elements work together to provide a thorough measurement of the quality of services provided. The next sections examine the three elements of a quality assurance program—structure, process, and outcome and follow with a discussion of their interrelationship.

Structure

Structure is the setting or framework under which the nurse–client relationship exists. It is the employing agency, *not* the home where the actual nurse–client interaction takes place. Structure includes

1. The philosophy or mission statement of an agency
2. The agency's objectives
3. Organizational structure of an agency
4. The agency's staffing patterns
5. Employment criteria for the agency
6. Available resources, such as equipment and supplies
7. The agency's communication patterns
8. Any other organizational characteristic of the agency (Wisnom, 1989)

Mission Statement. When evaluating the structure of an agency, one must begin by evaluating the mission statement or philosophy of the agency. What are the beliefs about the clients to be served and the type of nursing care to be delivered? For example, does the philosophy suggest that ill people cared for in the home are the primary clientele served by the agency? If so, is this consistent with the types of clients actually served by the agency? If the philosophy suggests that nursing care in the home is provided from a collaborative framework, does the agency employ other professionals and paraprofessionals to facilitate this collaboration? If nurses are expected to collaborate regularly with professionals outside the agency, are there adequate time and resources (telephone, secretarial support) to accomplish this objective? Examination of structure often involves looking for a match between what is written and what actually occurs within the agency.

Objectives. Following an examination of the mission statement or philosophy of an organization, evaluation of the agency objectives takes place. Agency objectives are statements of the goals of the agency. Often, agency philosophies are abstract in nature, including words and phrases that often do not have much meaning to the clinical practitioner. Objectives are used to translate into practice the intent of the mission statement or philosophy, from which they are derived. In evaluating the agency's stated objectives, the nurse tries to determine if the objectives of the organization are reflective of the stated beliefs identified in the philosophy. For example, if the philosophy suggests that the client is an active member of the heath care team, do the objectives reflect an active role for the client in the planning and implementation of care?

Organizational Structure and Staffing Patterns. The third and fourth areas of structural evaluation are examination of the organizational structure and staffing patterns of the agency. Both of these variables have a significant impact on the type and quality of nursing care provided. As discussed in chapter 1, the organizational structure of the agency can be identified by examining the agency's organizational chart. Line and staff relationships, as well as reporting mechanisms and supervisory relationships, can be identified. The staffing patterns, the methods used to recruit skilled employees and assign specific responsibilities within the agency, may not be readily identifiable from reading the organizational chart. It may be necessary to interview the individual responsible for hiring within the agency to determine the desired staffing pattern for the agency. In times of severe nursing shortages, the desired staffing pattern for the agency may be very different from the actual staffing pattern.

Employment Criteria. Another structural aspect, which must be evaluated in a quality assurance program, is made up of the agency's employment criteria. The employment criteria of the agency should be consistent with the role requirements of the nurses in the home care setting. For example, if the philosophy suggests that one of the roles of the nurses within the agency involves developing new nursing knowledge through research, the nurses hired by that agency should have the skills, either through experience or education, to conduct or participate in clinical nursing research. Similarly, if the agency uses a case manager approach, the nurses hired as case managers should possess the skills to function in that role.

Resources. Any resource, such as equipment or supplies, that the agency uses may be assessed as part of the structural evaluation, since adequacy of resources often affects client care directly. A resource can be defined as something as simple as a policy manual. Does the agency have a policy manual, and is there easy access to it by staff members? An agency that does not have enough stethoscopes for the nurses to use cannot expect nurses to take blood pressure measurements for their clients. In this situation, the quality of care the nurses can provide is directly affected by a structural aspect of an agency. Office supplies and resources are included in the evaluation of the structural aspects of an agency.

Communication Patterns. The communication patterns used throughout the agency form another structural aspect that must be assessed in a quality assurance program. In large health care agencies, many organizational problems can be attributed to inadequately developed communication systems. Home care agencies often face problems with communication, not because of their size, but because their staff members are independent in their practice and see each other to communicate on issues of concern infrequently. In these situations, written communications, such as memos, policy statements, and procedure instructions, are used to assure that all staff members concerned receive the same message. When evaluating the communication patterns within an agency, all forms of communication (e.g., memos, newsletters, announcements, verbal communication) must be considered. Assessment of the structural aspects of an agency provides the necessary foundation for the evaluation of the next two elements involved in quality assurance.

Process

Evaluation of the process aspect, or dimension, of the quality assurance program focuses exclusively on the activities of the nurse. Process is the sequence of events and activities of nursing care. It involves the clinical performance of the nurse including the degree of skill, the interactions between the nurse and the client, and the degree of client involvement in the care provided.

Assessment of the process dimension of quality assurance involves examination of the use of the nursing process to determine if it is used appropriately in working with clients and families. Process evaluation includes review of the activities carried out by the nurse, or her designee, in order to help clients meet their specific health care goals. It must be remembered that the process dimension not only examines the activities of the primary care nurse, it also involves the activities of all other professionals and paraprofessionals involved in the implementation of the interventions described in the client care plan. For example, evaluation of the process dimension in quality assurance involves reviewing the activities of the home health aide to determine if the services provided were appropriate, timely, and supervised by a professional.

There are many ways in which the information regarding the activities and events of nursing care can be measured. The most common type of process evaluation, the **nursing audit**, is defined as "a method of evaluating the quality of care through the appraisal of the nursing process as it is reflected in the patient care record" (Phaneuf, 1976, p. 32). Audits can be

retrospective or concurrent. A retrospective audit is done with records for clients who have been discharged from the agency. An evaluation of the total implementation of the nursing process can be made since the client has already received all care and has been discharged from the agency. Concurrent audits are done using charts of clients who are currently receiving care from the agency. These clients may be newly admitted to the agency or may be approaching discharge from home care services.

The chart is the central index of information of all aspects of client care and is, therefore, used for the audit. As such, charting is the most effective method of documenting and communicating all vital information. The chart becomes a reflection of the quality of care the client receives and the measure of the level of professional practice of the home care nurse. Since the chart is used to evaluate the quality of care a client receives, the importance of accurate and comprehensive documentation on the chart cannot be overemphasized.

A nursing audit is accomplished with the use of a nursing audit tool. This tool or instrument is developed by the agency and is based on the expected standards of care. When a chart is selected for review, usually at random, the nursing audit tool is used to provide the format for evaluation of all services provided. The reviewer examines what is documented in the record against the criteria detailed in the nursing audit instrument. An example of a specific criterion on a nursing audit instrument is "All nursing entries are signed." Using the nursing audit instrument, the chart is reviewed to determine if all nursing entries are signed by all the nurses who provided care to this client.

Audits may be internal or external. The internal audits are completed by other practicing nurses or supervisors employed by the agency who have not cared for the client directly. External audits are conducted by professionals, with, it is hoped, home care experience, who review the records of their disciplines using the same formalized audit tool. The external audit is felt to be an objective measure of process quality.

Since the nursing audit instrument provides the format used to appraise the implementation of the nursing process used with specific clients, it will be helpful for the nurse to examine the nursing audit instrument used in her agency. This will give the home care nurse an idea of the criteria used to evaluate a client record. A judgment regarding the quality of client care provided will be based only on what is written in the client care record; therefore, nursing audits reinforce the importance of accurate and complete documentation. If the record does not reflect that specific assessments, interventions, or evaluations were performed by the nurse, it will be assumed by the reviewer that they were not done. The record may indicate there were deficiencies in the care provided when in fact, the deficiencies were in the documentation of care.

Following the review of the record using the audit instrument, the reviewer will identify the next step in the auditing process. For example, if no major deficiencies and good work was found, there may be no further action taken on this record except to give positive feedback to the nurses involved. If there were minor deficiencies found in the record, the supervisor may discuss these with the specific nurse so that the nurse can improve the quality of her practice. If major deficiencies have been identified, the chart may have to be referred to a secondary review committee, which could make suggestions for policy decisions to avoid similar problems in the future. The process for determining to whom the chart will be referred following review is made by the agency and can be described by the nursing supervisor.

Another method of process evaluation is **supervisory evaluation of staff performance**. Most likely, in addition to reading the nurse's clinical records and having case conferences, the supervisor will want to make joint visits with the home care nurse to evaluate directly the nursing care being provided to clients in the home. This is a useful learning experience for the new staff nurse since the supervisor will be able to give feedback on the care provided and evaluate the nurse's charting based on that home visit. It is important that the nurse view this joint visit as an opportunity to improve her clinical practice skills. The nurse should be open to the suggestions and constructive criticism made by the supervisor. The nursing supervisor's role is to discuss different perspectives and approaches to the delivery of care to clients and not to be punitive in her judgments.

Soliciting information from the client can also supply data for the assessment of care provided by the nurse. A face-to-face interview with the client can be conducted to ask such questions as "What did you like about the nursing care you received?" or "Were there specific problems with the care you received?" This technique is not used often because, many times, the client is not the best judge of how effectively the nursing process was utilized to meet the identified health needs. As a nonprofessional, the client is unable to evaluate the subtle aspects of professional practice that are essential parts of quality care.

In addition to face-to-face interviews, nonidentifying surveys and questionnaires can be sent out by the agency. Although the information obtained through surveys and questionnaires can be useful, often this method of collecting quality assurance data suffers some problems with thoroughness. The clients who respond tend to be either very happy with the care provided or extremely dissatisfied. Therefore, the agency only obtains data reflective of very positive or very negative perceptions. A second problem with surveys is that clients may not be totally honest in their responses if they feel that they could be identified by their responses in some way. Even if there is little identifying information requested on the questionnaire, people may respond in a socially acceptable manner. As a result, the data obtained from clients need to be evaluated and utilized with a recognition of the problems inherent in this data collection strategy.

When assessing the process dimension of the quality assurance program, which is focused on the activities of the nurse, often there is a great deal of anxiety on the part of both the evaluator of care and the nurse whose record is being evaluated. The evaluator, either from within the agency or outside, often feels anxious about identifying deficiencies on the record of a colleague or even a friend. Although it may be difficult to review a colleague's records, it must be remembered that peer evaluation is part of the role of a professional. Also, it must be remembered that a nursing audit is done for the purpose of improving the quality of care that clients receive, not for the purpose of identifying individual staff weaknesses. The outcome of process evaluation often focuses on identification of staff strengths rather than individual nurses' weaknesses.

Outcome

The third phase of a quality assurance program centers on the assessment of outcomes. The outcome dimension of the quality assurance model program focuses on assessing the measured change in the client's behavior as it relates to the care provided. Outcome measures examine the end results of nursing care and measure behavioral changes in the client rather than examine the process used by the nurse to effect that client change. For example, an outcome criterion might be "the client will be able to instill his own eye drops using appropriate technique." In order to evaluate this criterion, the nurse would determine if the client can perform this procedure, which is the outcome of care. The evaluator would not be concerned about **how** the client learned this appropriate technique for instilling eye drops but rather would evaluate the client's ability to perform the designated procedure.

In order to measure outcomes, basic criteria must be defined. These criteria are developed from the standards of care and identify behaviors that the client should achieve as a result of nursing intervention.

Criteria are measurable statements that reflect the intent of a standard and relate to specific diseases that will be encountered in home care practice. For example, a standard for a client with COPD might be, "The client will remain free from exacerbation of illness." This general statement needs some measurable criteria to make it meaningful to the practitioner. Criteria for a client with COPD might include the following:

- The client's temperature will remain within normal limits.
- The client will be able to identify a low-sodium diet and plan nutritious meals within those parameters.
- The client will be able to plan his activities of daily living, integrating rest periods with necessary activity.
- The client's significant other will be knowledgeable regarding the prescribed care regime for the client.

The behaviors of the client with COPD at discharge would be evaluated against these identified criteria as one way to evaluate the care provided.

Some home care agencies choose not to base their outcome measures on criteria related to specific diseases but rather to identify an overall goal of client care and evaluate client outcomes based on that goal. Client classification systems have been developed to measure changes in client behaviors based on level of dependence or ability for self-management. For example, a home care agency might identify independence as the goal of client care for their agency. This would first be reflected in the philosophy or mission statement for that particular agency (structure). Nursing care would focus on those activities that foster independence in clients (process). The agency would then identify the criteria that relate to independence. Client behaviors at discharge would be evaluated against those identified criteria (outcome). Since these criteria would not relate to a specific disease, they could be used to evaluate all client outcomes, regardless of the diagnosis. Examples of "independence" criteria could include the following:

- The client will be able to perform his activities of daily living without assistance.
- The client will have the necessary skills and possess sufficient knowledge to manage his medical care regime.
- The client will identify those areas where support is needed from others and secure that assistance.

Interrelationship of Structure, Process, and Outcome

Once data have been collected on the structure, process, and outcome aspects of care, interpretations must be made about the quality of care provided. This is the most important element of quality assurance, since it is through this evaluative process that suggestions for change and improvement are made in various areas of the agency. The strengths of the nursing staff can also be identified through this evaluative process.

It is important to remember that quality of care cannot be evaluated through the examination of only *one* phase of the quality assurance model program. For example, by examining only the process aspect, which focuses on the activities of the nurse, the evaluator will learn valuable information regarding the implementation of the nursing process but will not be able to determine the effectiveness of those interventions on the client's behaviors. Similarly, by examining only the outcome aspect of the quality assurance model, one would be able to evaluate the changes in the client's behaviors but would lack information about the nursing activities that assisted in that change (Carron, 1988).

Every nurse has experienced a situation in which a client would not modify his or her behaviors to reflect the teaching that was done. Regardless of the interventions performed with this client, the behaviors did not reflect the amount of time, energy, and expertise put into the client's care. By evaluating the outcomes only, the evaluator may suggest that the care provided was deficient. After evaluation of the process and outcome elements, the evaluator would see that the nursing process was implemented appropriately and that the client outcomes were not a result of inadequate nursing care.

In summary, quality assurance has always been a concern of nurses and the nursing profession. Factors within the nursing profession, such as standards of care, and pressures from outside the profession, such as third party payors, have combined to focus increased attention on quality assurance in home care nursing. A typical method of assessing quality of care is through the examination of the structure, process, and outcomes elements of nursing practice. The interrelationship of structure, process, and outcome in the evaluation of the quality of nursing care provided cannot be overemphasized. Examination of all three aspects is essential to provide the evaluator and the agency with an accurate picture of the quality of care provided.

TEST YOURSELF

1. Identify four charting principles that must be kept in mind when recording in a home care record.

2. Identify the five criteria that a client must meet to be eligible for home care services under Medicare. Define each in your own words.

3. Complete form 485 and form 486 for a client you visited during your orientation period. Review it with your supervisor.

4. Review the mission statement or philosophy of your agency to determine the types of clients served and the roles and responsibilities of the home care nurse.

5. Review the objectives of your agency to see if there is congruence between what is written in the philosophy and the stated objectives.

6. Examine the organizational chart for your agency. See if you can identify the relationships between members of the organization. For example, who is your immediate supervisor? To whom does your supervisor report? To whom does the executive director (CEO) report?

7. Review the employment criteria for your agency. Are employment criteria for specific agency positions identified?

8. Try to identify all the methods used by your agency to obtain information about the process aspects of the quality assurance process.

9. Review the outcome measure instrument used by your agency. Do you feel comfortable writing outcomes based on your agency's system? How are client outcomes evaluated? And by whom?

Strategies for Effective Clinical Management

OBJECTIVES

Upon completion of this chapter the reader will be able to identify

1. The ways a home care nursing department can be organized
2. A definition of case load management
3. Ways to be more efficient in home care nursing practice
4. Criteria for determining frequency of visits
5. Phases of contracting in home care
6. Steps of the teaching–learning process
7. The application of teaching–learning principles to home care clients
8. Items necessary to document client teaching

KEY CONCEPTS

- **How a home care nurse fits into a nursing unit**

- **How to work smarter, not harder**

- **Determining when a client needs visits**

- **Setting up realistic expectations with clients**

- **Various approaches to client teaching**

AGENCY-SPECIFIC MATERIAL NEEDED

- Tickler card/client monitoring system used to plan visits
- Route slips
- Time sheets
- Productivity standards and ways of evaluating productivity
- Teaching aids available for client distribution
- Standardized teaching flowsheets
- Blank client care record (for exercise)

HOME CARE NURSING DELIVERY STRATEGIES

The importance of the staff nurse's understanding of the organizational structure and function of the total agency early in her orientation was discussed in chapter 1. Once that understanding takes place, it is then essential that discussion focus on the organization of the nursing department or unit within the agency. Since nursing plays the pivotal role in a home health agency, the nursing department should be organized so that work is carried out effectively and efficiently and that the nurse is supported in the tasks she performs caring for clients.

This chapter explores organizational models of nursing units with the sections that follow covering the related subjects of case load and work load management, productivity, time management, and contracting; all crucial aspects to effective home care nursing. Following these sections, patient teaching, an essential component of home care nursing practice, is discussed. This chapter, reviewed in light of the nursing process applied to home care outlined in chapter 2 forms the base of the home care nurse's practice and allows the nurse to function at her highest level in the agency.

Organizational Models for Nursing Units

All nurses are familiar with the standard models of nursing care delivery—primary, functional, team, and case method—based on their student or work experiences. These models are used in home care agencies but often with different objectives, since homecare is provided outside an institution and is a more independent practice. The various delivery models will be presented, outlining the way(s) they are used in a home health agency. It is important to remember that these models focus solely on the responsibilities of nursing personnel in an agency—registered professional nurses (RNs) and licensed vocational nurses (LVNs). Client care activities carried out by paraprofessionals, such as home health aides (HHAs), are always directly supervised by the nurse conducting the home visit or the primary care nurse. It is the responsibility of the nurse in charge of the case in the specific nursing model outlined to develop the care plan and supervise all home health aide care given to a client. Home health aide supervision is covered more extensively in chapter 5.

Primary Care Nursing. Primary nursing combines the concepts of total client care and all-professional nursing staff. In primary nursing, a registered nurse (the *primary* nurse) assumes total responsibility for planning the care of one or more clients from admission to the agency to discharge. The primary nurse estab-

lishes the care plan and provides direct care for clients assigned to her. If someone else provides care in her absence, those providers follow the care plan established by the primary nurse and report back to her. It is also the responsibility of the primary nurse to coordinate communication between all members of the health care team and the client and family. Good communication and feedback are essential when primary nursing is the model used in a home health agency.

In home care, the primary care nursing model has been used extensively, but increasing costs and the decreasing availability of registered nurses have made this model difficult to implement in an environment that regulates costs so strictly. Often the model is used in combination with the team approach, in which RNs are seen as the individual primary nurses and LVNs are supervised as part of the team and work under the direction of the RNs.

Team Nursing. In team nursing, small groups of nurses work together as a team under the direction of a professional nurse called a team leader. As coordinator of the team, the team leader is responsible for knowing about and planning the care of each client cared for by her team regardless of whether she directly cares for the client. In team nursing, communication between members is essential and can be achieved by formal methods, such as team conferences held on a periodic basis, or informal methods, such as having the team leader communicate frequently with team members.

Team nursing has been used successfully by many home health agencies. By using highly trained and experienced home care nurses to lead the team and make client assignments, RN and LVN team members can contribute their own special skills in caring for clients. For example, if a member of a team is especially apt at caring for clients with ostomies, then she might care of the majority of the team's clients with this condition. Some agencies that use team nursing have the team leader visit clients and perform supervisory functions for the members of her team. The team leader coordinates the care given to all clients, and other members of the team are kept up-to-date on the progress of the team's clients at team meetings and conferences. It is important to remember that in team nursing, all team members share the responsibility and accountability for the nursing care delivered.

Functional Nursing. Functional nursing, historically seen as the most economical means of providing care, is the model that assigns specific tasks to the nurse, rather than one that delegates total care of specific patients to an individual nurse. For example, a medication nurse, treatment nurse, and charge nurse are roles assumed by nurses in hospitals to perform certain functions, and on a unit all three nurses, each with a different role, could be carrying out the various tasks for the same patient during a shift. Since it would be ineffective and inefficient to have various nurses see an individual client in their home, functional nursing is not a model used to provide home care services.

Case Method. The case method model of nursing, or total patient care, is the oldest model of organizing client care. This model was used at the turn of the 19th century by private duty nurses who delivered care primarily in the client's home. Today the model is used primarily in intensive care settings within an acute hospital. The true case method model of nursing is not used in home care agencies, although one could argue that it is used if a client only has a private duty nurse, which might be hired through another branch of the agency (Marquis & Huston, 1987).

Case Management. In the late 1980s, case management and managed care became the buzzwords of health care delivery. New case management models are evolving in institutional and outpatient settings. Some home health agencies have organized their nursing units using a case management model; often this model varies somewhat among agencies and may be a combination of the models discussed so far. The discussion of case management and managed care, which follows this section, will help to clarify the different ways that case management can function in a home care nursing department and the roles that nurses can assume in the models.

Some home health agencies implement the case management model, in which the case manager (CM) functions as a team leader and directs the care given to a group of clients (team nursing). The CM may also provide direct care to a group of clients (primary care) and assume supervisory responsibilities, such as the orientation of staff, development of management reports, and evaluation of staff members who work under their supervision. In this model the case manager tracks the reimbursement of clients but does not formally evaluate and report the cost-effectiveness of the care given.

Managed Care. The home care nurse must understand that there are other definitions of the terms case management and managed care that will be encountered as she works with clients, other providers, and payment sources outside the agency. The discussion of nursing models above addressed case management as a model to organize nursing services in a home health agency. There are other definitions and

models of case management, which will be described briefly. Desimone (1988, p. 22) defines case management as a systematic approach to

- Identifying high-risk/high-cost patients
- Assessing opportunities to coordinate care
- Assessing and choosing treatment options
- Developing treatment plans to improve quality and efficacy
- Controlling costs
- Managing a patient's total care to ensure optimum outcome

The nature and objectives of case management models may vary, depending on the organizational structure of the system and whether the system is linked to reimbursement. Case management may be provided by health care facilities, insurance companies, social agencies, health maintenance organizations (HMOs), or private companies. Various professionals may assume the role of case manager. For example, a primary care physician might be the person designated to approve a plan of care or an allied health or nonmedical professional, such as a social worker, might act as a case manager. Nurses have also assumed various case management functions in the different models.

Managed care has been defined by Victor Cohn (1988, p. 22), as having five parts:

- Preadmission certification of any proposed hospitalization
- Concurrent review, meaning a reviewer continues to monitor hospitalization
- Case management or individual benefits management, meaning the managers will strongly suggest cheaper alternatives to long hospital stays
- Second opinions
- Bonuses or penalties for the physician depending upon the cost of care

Knollmueller (1989, p. 38) defines case management as a process more than a structure or outcome. She goes on to discuss the American Nurses' Association description of nursing case management as "... a healthcare delivery process whose goals are to provide quality healthcare, decrease fragmentation, enhance the client's quality of life and contain costs." This coordination of care and communication with all care providers is what public health and home care nurses have been doing for years.

Although managed care and case management are often used synonymously, based on the discussions presented previously, they are very different. In most situations, the term case management describes the coordination of care a client receives within the context of the benefit system, but not directly linked to, the payor of services. In other words, the case manager considers the care a person needs but is not totally responsible for finding all the payment sources to pay for the needed care. In some instances, case managers and case management systems are set up independently of direct care providers so that the risk of conflict of interest in minimized. Managed care, on the other hand, is the coordination of client services administered by the payor of services, such as an insurance company. Managed care is always tied to reimbursement and the systems developed to oversee the care provided are linked to payment and utilization of services. For example, an insurance company may have a managed care department that will look for cost effective ways of caring for clients with certain diseases. That department, then, authorizes the care given in light of the client's insurance benefits and the least expensive services needed to reach the client's goals.

PRODUCTIVITY

Increasing concern about health care costs and the need to control factors that improve efficiency have increased the focus on productivity in home health agencies. The discussion of productivity and visit standards need not conjure up negative responses from staff members within an agency if everyone understands the reasons why productivity and visit standards are so important to a home health agency. First, no agency can survive without at least breaking even on expenses and income, and to do that, personnel must be efficient. Second, the agency wants to assure quality, and monitoring productivity can increase the likelihood that staff members are providing high-quality care.

Although productivity is difficult to measure in health care, it is not impossible, and many home health agencies have developed ways to reach this goal. Before the home care nurse can become familiar with the productivity standards used in an agency and understand how they are applied, she must understand the following productivity concepts summarized here from Benefield's (1988) work:

- Productivity is the relationship between the use of resources and the results of that use.
- Efficiency is not necessarily how fast work is done, but how well time is used.
- Quality can improve at the same time that productivity increases.
- Improving productivity involves all departments in a home health agency, never just one department or staff.
- Productivity is a "people issue," and since approximately 80% of a home health agency's budget is

spent on personnel, *all* agency personnel contribute to productivity.
- Hands on skills are very important, but so also is the home care nurse's ability to think critically, solve problems, and make decisions that impact on the total care the client receives. These attributes must be factored into productivity issues.
- Visit standards should be developed that consider the intensity of service provided to the client (complexity level of the client), and the case mix (types of clients) of the population served by the agency. They should also take into consideration the efficiency of the paperflow in the total organization.
- Effectiveness of the service is an important productivity component and a crucial aspect of the agency's quality assurance program. The expectations of the outcomes of the home visit as well as the standards set for what is to go on in a home visit are important parts of understanding productivity in home care.

Factors That Affect Productivity

A staff nurse should be constantly looking for ways to work smarter, not harder. Studies of the professional productivity conclude that the focus should not be on working faster (rushing through visits) but on using time efficiently and spending time doing those skills that the nurse was trained to do (Benefield, 1988). This is an important concept for all employees of the agency to remember, and it can be helpful when finding ways to help others be more efficient. There are several factors that can be considered to increase productivity.

Case Load Management. The case load is a group of clients assigned. For a primary nurse, a case manager, or a team leader, the case load will be the clients whose care she must direct. As a member of a team, the case load will be the case(s) assigned for a given time period, such as a day, week, or whatever the length of time the client is on service. The way that the work relating to these clients is organized is termed case load management.

There are many factors that affect the nurse's ability to manage a case load including

1. The frequency (number of times a week) and length (visit time) of visits to the case load clients
2. The specific needs of the clients in the case load (i.e., teaching, direct care, coordinating multi-agency involvement, and psychosocial involvement). This can be visit- or nonvisit-related time
3. The level of difficulty of the clients in your case load. This is usually determined by a client classification system used in the agency that categorizes

the level of acuity experienced by clients using several different variables

Each agency should have systems in place to help the nurse to learn skills of case load management. The best resources for learning case load management are scheduling conferences with a supervisor about client issues and working with experienced nurses who can share the ways they have found to be more efficient. Also, by using the strategies outlined in the home visiting section of Chapter 2, and the suggestions listed in the following pages about contracting and patient teaching, the nurse will be able to develop her case load management skills.

Work Load Management. Work load is a summary of all the activities of a home care nurse, including case load management. Each agency should have a process for analyzing a nurse's work load often through the use of forms to be completed or interactions with the nursing supervisor. In addition to the material collected for measuring the case load management activities, the nurse will be recording the time spent on activities other than home visiting. These can include agency activities such as in-service programs, staff meetings, and conferences; community activities such as clinics or committee work; work in off-site areas such as schools; and personal time such as lunch, holidays, and vacations.

The new staff nurse may not be familiar with keeping track of her daily time in this manner. She should be assured that she is asked to do this, not because of agency distrust, but because the nature of home care is independent, and the agency needs to collect this information to justify costs to regulatory bodies and for budgeting purposes. Federal agencies, such as the Internal Revenue Service and the Social Security Administration, also require that this information be recorded. It is important that this information be accurate and up-to-date to be fair to the nurse and the agency.

Time Management. The only manager of a home care nurse's time is the nurse. To be effective and efficient in professional practice, the nurse must be insightful concerning her use of time. The new home care nurse will identify many items that are time-wasters or time-savers, adding to the list that may have been started earlier in her career. Home care is a very independent practice, and the nurse must use self-discipline and motivation to stay efficient. The use of contracting, outlined in this chapter is the best time-saver a home care nurse can use in clinical practice working directly with clients. There are other ways to manage time effectively and they are listed below.

- Schedule clients who live in close proximity to each other together to minimize travel time.
- Keep a daily file to identify clients that need to be seen and other activities planned for certain days. A tickler card file or a calendar appointment book can be used to keep information from becoming misplaced. This is important so that planned visits are kept track of, and clients are seen on time.
- Find a quiet place to do your recording. This is not always easy in a small office that has a lot of distracting activity going on. If possible, documentation should be completed in the client's home during the visit or immediately after the visit. Many nurses find restaurants in their visiting area that offer enough space and privacy to do their paperwork while the nurse has a soft drink or cup of coffee. If most of the nurse's visit recording is completed before her return to the office, she will be better prepared for the other work activities that await her and the quality of the recording will improve because the information will have been recorded when it was clear in her memory.
- Charting should be done so well that few additional notes are needed. The recording should be complete enough that if there must be communication with others, such as social workers or physical therapists, the client's record should include the bulk of the required information. Nurses are notorious for repeating orally what they have written (or should have written) in the record—a carry over from the change-of-shift report. This is a waste of time, especially in home care.
- Limit socializing. Most of the workday is spent with clients not colleagues, so it is important to make time to socialize with coworkers. The nurse must determine when that will be and for how long. Meeting with other nurses for lunch can often be a positive use of time while it frees up the time in the office for work-related issues.
- Keep phone time to a minimum. Make all telephone calls in one block of time as much as possible, and always have something to work on (e.g., a client record) while on hold. Prepare an agenda for phone conversations to avoid forgetting any pieces of information.
- Delegate work to others. The agency employs support staff that are available to free the nurse up for nursing-related functions. The staff nurse should look for ways to improve the quality of interaction among agency staff members, through constructive feedback to the supervisor and in staff meetings. Remember, when a nurse identifies a problem area it is up to her also to develop ways to solve it and then become committed to making the approach work.
- Always call clients and give them an approximate

time for the home visit (e.g., late morning, early afternoon). Do not predict a precise arrival time since scheduling is based on estimated time spent on earlier visits, and the nurse does not want to set up a situation where the patient is worried needlessly about the nurse because she is 15 minutes late.

- Always put specific directions to the client's home on the record so that finding the way will be easier for the nurse and other staff members who may visit the client.

DETERMINING FREQUENCY OF VISITS

Determining how often a client is visited, and when the next visit following admission needs to be scheduled, often is the responsibility of the home care nurse. In collaboration with the physician, the home care nurse must determine if the client needs daily, biweekly, weekly, or monthly home visits. The condition of the client and any agency, state or federal policies are significant variables in determining how often a client will receive home visits. The following section provides a guideline that can be used by the home care nurse to determine the frequency of home visits (Humphrey, 1986). The nurse must remember that clients come to home care with complex problems that require careful monitoring and skilled intervention. Considering the combination of complex situations, it would be impossible for the home care nurse to collect all necessary data to develop a complete plan of care and perform the skilled necessary interventions on the first visit to a client's home. Consequently, for most clients, an admission visit and a second visit scheduled fairly close together (within 1 or 2 days) will be necessary in order to develop a complete and accurate care plan. Reasons why home care nurses might schedule home visits at the following intervals are listed below.

Next Day Visits

- The nurse has an incomplete data base on which to make a judgment and needs to obtain more data the next day.
- The client has an immediate teaching need, which cannot be completed on the first visit.
- The client's condition is unstable and likely to change in the period of a day.
- The client's plan of care involves a complex technical procedure that requires the skill of a professional nurse.
- The family is having serious difficulty coping with the care of the client at home and needs guidance and direction.

- A significant other who can help with the care of the client has not been identified.

Next Visit in 2 or 3 Days

- The nurse is monitoring a client who is progressing toward independence.
- The care provided by a significant other who has the primary responsibility for the skilled intervention is being evaluated.
- The evaluation of the effectiveness of the teaching that was done with the client and family is conducted. The nurse continues to implement the teaching plan and reinforce the teaching that was previously accomplished.
- The client's plan of care involves biweekly skilled intervention (e.g., decubitus care with duoderm).
- The nurse is evaluating the effectiveness of a treatment plan.

Weekly Visits

- The client is approaching independence but must be monitored one last time before discharge.
- The client's plan of care involves a weekly skilled intervention (e.g., changing an Unna boot).
- The nurse must evaluate the coping abilities of the family as the client approaches discharge.
- The client needs minimal monitoring.
- The nurse must perform a specific intervention (e.g., pre-fill insulin syringes).

Monthly Visits

- The client has achieved the optimal level of functioning.
- The client's plan of care involves monthly skilled intervention (e.g., vitamin B_{12} injection).
- The nurse must satisfy regulations or compliance with reimbursement guidelines.

CONTRACTING IN HOME CARE

One of the significant functions to be performed by a home care nurse is the promotion of healthy behaviors through the identification of client needs and the development of plans to meet those needs. The client's active participation in the assessment and planning phase of the therapeutic relationship has been shown to be effective in helping the client to learn and practice healthy behaviors. Contracting can be used by the home care nurse to promote the active role of the client in all phases of the nursing process. This section includes a description of the concept of contracting, followed by a description of the phases of the contracting process. A discussion of the advantages of contracting in the home care setting concludes this section.

The Concept of Contracting

Contracting is defined as any working agreement between the nurse and the client that is continually being renegotiated (Sloan & Schommer, 1982). It is an agreement between the client and the nurse that provides the framework for planning and evaluating the interactions that are occurring. It accomplishes this by identifying what each person in the relationship can expect from the other person in the relationship—what behaviors the nurse can expect from the client and what behaviors the client can expect from the nurse.

The concept of legal contracts is familiar to everyone. Nursing contracts differ in that they are not legally binding and are much more flexible than legal contracts. Contracts are used primarily to increase the role played by the client in the health care process. Through the identification and formalization of the client's role in the individual health care plan, the cooperative relationship between the nurse and the client strengthens.

There are eight steps in the process of contracting. Both nurse and client have significant responsibilities in each step of the process, mandating active involvement of both parties through the entire process. The eight steps of contracting in nursing are

- Exploration of a need
- Establishment of goals
- Exploration of resources
- Development of a plan
- Division of responsibilities
- Agreement on a time frame
- Evaluation
- Renegotiation or termination

Each one of these steps of the contracting process will be discussed in detail.

Phases of the Contracting Process

Contracting is a learned process between the nurse and the client. All parties must have an understanding of the process of contracting for this strategy to be effective. Sloan and Schommer (1982) describe eight phases that make up the contracting process.

1. **Exploration of need.** This phase involves the assessment by both the client and the nurse of the client's health needs and problems. Identification of the client's perspective regarding his health status and his treatment plan is an essential component of this first phase.

2. **Establishment of goals.** Through discussion, the nurse and the client establish mutually agreeable goals for the purpose of alleviating the identified health problem or need. Goals should be realistic and attainable; the tendency to set overly ambitious goals should be avoided. Goals should be recognized as dynamic, which means that they can be renegotiated if they are unrealistic or are no longer relevant.

3. **Exploration of resources.** In this phase, the nurse and the client define how each can contribute to achieving the identified health goal. The nurse and the client should work together to identify appropriate resources, such as significant others, community services, and other professionals, that can play a role in alleviating the identified health need.

4. **Development of a plan.** Activities designed to meet the specified goals are developed in this phase of the process. If there is more than one goal, the nurse and the client collaborate to develop a priority list of identified goals. Identifying activities to meet one goal at a time, beginning with the one with the highest priority, prevents the client from feeling overwhelmed by the contracting process and the implementation of the plan.

5. **Division of responsibilities.** In this phase, the nurse and the client decide who will be responsible for which activities. At first, the client may feel fearful in assuming activities identified as the professional responsibility of the nurse. As a client experiences success in managing his or her situation, the client will feel more at ease in assuming greater responsibility for his or her own health care.

6. **Agreement on a time frame.** As in all areas of goal setting and intervention, a time frame for accomplishment of goals must be determined. At the initial visit, the home care nurse should work with the client to develop a plan that outlines the anticipated frequency of home visits based on doctor's orders and the nursing assessment. This planning is conducted in all agencies, and nurses are required to complete this for various forms and for their own case management plans; often, however, nurses do not share this important information with the client. For example, the home care nurse, in collaboration with the client, might plan to make home visits three times per week for 2 weeks, two times per week for 2 weeks, and then one time per week for 4 weeks. Both client and nurse should agree on the established time frame and the specific goals to be accomplished at each step of the 8-week period. By doing this, both the

client and the nurse know what is expected and how they are progressing on the goals developed.

7. **Evaluation.** Assessment of progress toward the goals or accomplishment of the goals is done in this phase. The nurse and the client evaluate the progress to date, both in terms of the client outcomes and the interventions used to facilitate that outcome.

8. **Renegotiation or termination.** Based on the evaluation, the nurse and the client determine if the contract needs to be renegotiated or terminated. If the goal has been met, the contract can be terminated. If the goal has not been met, the contract can be modified and renegotiated. Any part of the contract may require modification. Perhaps the goals were too ambitious or the interventions inappropriate to meet the designated goal. In some cases, the nurse may have to assume tasks previously assigned to the client with the client assuming responsibility for other activities. Different strategies can be tried before contracting is abandoned.

Nursing contracts can be formal or informal, depending on how comfortable the nurse is with this intervention strategy, the client's readiness to assume responsibility for self-care, and the agency's policy. Formal contracts between the nurse and the client involve **written identification** of goals, including each person's responsibility in achievement of the goals, and signature of the written document by both parties. Less formal contracts, often used in home care situations, involve **verbal identification** of goals and each party's responsibility in achieving those goals are outlined. In an informal contract, the nurse and the client develop a plan and come to an oral understanding regarding each party's responsibility in the contract. Client goals and the methods selected for achieving them, then documented in the nursing care plan, form the written evidence for implementation and evaluation of how the contract was achieved. Contracting takes time and effort on the part of the nurse and the client, but it is more than worth the time and work required at the beginning of the home care nursing relationship.

Some clients are afraid to assume an active role in their health care. If a client does not feel ready to take an active role, contracting may not be an appropriate strategy to use at the onset of care. Some clients prefer to relinquish all power to the professional involved in their care. These clients tend to be passive recipients rather than active participants in their health care. Clients with minimal cognitive abilities often find difficulty with the concept of contracting. There must be an appreciation of the concept of commitment in order for contracting to constitute an effective intervention strategy.

In some cases, the home care nurse can persuade a hesitant client to accept the process of contracting. Through an explanation of the process, the client may see that contracting is not as difficult as it may sound. Clients may also be persuaded to try contracting if they know that they can get out of the contract at any step in the process. Unlike legal contracts, there is no binding effect to the nursing contract. Clients may also be persuaded to try contracting when it is described as a means to attaining their health care goals quickly and efficiently. In today's climate of cost containment and reimbursement limits, contracting is a useful tool in moving both the client and the nurse to the identified goal in an efficient manner.

The role of the nurse in the nurse–client relationship will be altered when employing the concept of contracting. The nurse must be willing to relinquish her control as the powerful expert. In a hospital, the nurse is usually in control of care and the patient is a passive recipient. In home care, the nurse and the client share equal authority in the relationship. The concept of contracting involves empowerment of the client, a concept that may frighten some professionals.

Contracting is most effective when there exists the potential for a long-term nursing relationship (more than two visits) between the client and the care provider. It is difficult to work through all the steps of the contracting process in one or two visits. As the nurse becomes adept at the contracting process and the client becomes accustomed to playing an active role in his or her health care, the contracting process can be accomplished in a shorter period of time.

In summary, contracting involves the active participation of the client and the nurse in the planning, implementation, and evaluation of the nursing care provided. This care centers on a common goal, with interventions geared toward the achievement of that goal. Contracts can be formal or as seen most commonly in home care, informal.

Benefits of contracting for the client and the nurse include the following:

- Time is saved in the long run by setting up a contract with the client at the onset of care.

- Contracting allows everyone, especially the client, to know what is going to happen and the timetable on which it is going to happen. This gives the client a sense of security. The client will know how long he or she will be receiving services and have an estimate of what the current goals are.

- Contracting keeps the nursing process goal directed and focused, thereby increasing the likelihood of reimbursement by third party payors such as Medicare, Medicaid, or private insurance.

Advantages of Contracting in Home Care

There are several reasons why contracting is an important intervention strategy in the practice of home care nursing. First, by the development of a plan through contracting, the roles and expectations of the nurse and the client become clarified. Increased clarity often enhances the nurse–client relationship. When each person is aware of his or her role and responsibility in the therapeutic relationship, the chance of meeting designated goals effectively increases.

Second, in home care nursing the relationship between the client and family and the nurse in unlike that seen in an inpatient facility, such as a hospital. In the hospital, the nurse assumes the responsibility for providing for the majority of care given to clients. In the home, the home care nurse's role is to teach the client or family member how to provide the necessary care to improve or maintain the client's level of health. The nature of the care delivery system dictates that clients and families play an active role in the health care provided. Contracting is a process in which that active role is given due recognition.

Other advantages to using contracting in the home care setting include

- The client plays an active role in his health care, rather than remaining a passive recipient of the care provided.
- Client empowerment and self-esteem are increased as success is experienced in self-care.
- New sets of coping strategies and decision-making skills are developed for the client.
- The possibility of achieving health goals identified by the client and the nurse increases because all parties are clear about the goal to be reached.
- Clearly defined goals, made achievable in measurable terms, can be used to motivate a client toward achievement of those goals.
- Increased focus on the interventions and evaluation of the intervention is possible, thereby increasing the likelihood of reimbursement by third party payors.

Again, in summary, contracting is an intervention strategy in which the nurse and the client (1) identify goals, (2) determine activities to achieve those goals, (3) identify who will assume responsibility for accomplishing those activities, and (4) evaluate the achievement of the goal. Contracts between clients and home care nurses can be very formal, with all steps to the process written with signatures of each party on the written document. More commonly, contracts are informal, oral agreements in which each step of the process is negotiated between the nurse and the client, and an oral evaluation is used to measure attainment of the goal.

CLIENT TEACHING

It is widely recognized that one of the many professional roles of the nurse involves client education. In home care nursing, this responsibility is even more pressing due to the limited number of visits with the client and family and because the major responsibility for the health care of the client rests with someone other than the nurse. Client education is one of the three components that Medicare considers skilled service and is, therefore, reimbursable. The other two skilled services that Medicare considers reimbursable are direct care services and observation, and assessment of the client's condition. Home care nurses have identified client education as being frequently underutilized and underdocumented in practice (Jackson & Johnson, 1988). It is imperative that home care nurses gain a working knowledge of the teaching–learning process and be able to implement it with clients and families in the home setting.

The teaching–learning process, like the nursing process, can be examined in terms of the activities that occur at each step of the process. This section explores the teaching–learning process, in general, followed by an assessment of learner readiness. This section also examines teaching intervention strategies and the process for evaluating teaching strategies used, and includes specific examples and illustrations.

Many students have sat through an in-service program or a class in nursing school and listened to a presenter for a period of time and realized when the presentation was finished that they had no idea what the instructor had been trying to teach. That is an important lesson about the teaching–learning process. Although the goal of all teaching is learning, very often the instructor and the student fall short of this goal. The process of giving information does not ensure that learning has taken place.

Learning occurs when a person is able to do something he or she was not able to do before. The home care nurse is involved in client education that has the potential to change some aspect of the client's behavior. The nurse can never assume that teaching alone will result in a behavior change. Clients, making choices about their health, may choose to continue unhealthy behaviors, even if they have the knowledge of why they should change and have the means to do so. In order to understand the teaching–learning process, the three forms of learning will be reviewed briefly.

The three forms of learning, as described by Bloom (1969) include the cognitive, affective, and psychomotor domains. The **cognitive domain** deals with "recall or recognition of knowledge and the development of individual abilities and skills"

(Bloom, 1969, p. 7). There are six major categories in the cognitive domain, including

- Knowledge. Recalling facts, methods, and procedures
- Comprehension. Combining recall and understanding to grasp the meaning of information.
- Application. Using information in new, specific, or concrete situations
- Analysis. Distinguishing between parts of information and understanding the relationship between them
- Synthesis. Putting the parts of information together in a unified whole
- Evaluation. Judging the value of ideas, procedures, and methods by using the appropriate criteria (Stanhope & Lancaster, 1988)

These categories form a hierarchy based on the degree of difficulty of the tasks at the various levels of learning. For example, a learner must know the four basic food groups (knowledge) before he or she can develop a balanced meal plan for the day (application). Similarly, a client must be able to follow a prescribed meal plan, including the four food groups (application), before he or she is able to substitute different foods on a basic exchange list (analysis).

The second domain as described by Bloom is the **affective domain**. This kind of learning involves "changes in interests, attitudes, values and the development of appreciations and adequate adjustment" (Bloom, 1969, p. 7). Although not as obvious as learning in the cognitive domain, nurses are frequently involved in the teaching–learning process in the affective domain. For example, the nurse who spends time during each visit discussing with the diabetic client the value of wearing slippers instead of going barefoot is teaching in the affective domain. The purpose of this teaching is to change the client's attitude toward going barefoot with a resultant change in behavior toward wearing slippers.

Affective learning occurs at several levels, depending on the learner's involvement and commitment. The levels include

- **Level 1** The learner is willing to listen and be attentive. For example, a home care nurse was working with a client, teaching the importance of diet in the client's recovery from coronary bypass surgery. On the first visit, the client was very interested in hearing what the nurse had to say and asked questions.
- **Level 2.** The learner becomes an active participant in the process. Based on the previous example, on the second visit the nurse found that the patient had completed a diet history and had had a friend purchase a copy of the *American Heart Association Cookbook*. Evaluating this behavior, the nurse deter-

mined that the client had become an active participant in the learning and was not just listening passively.
- **Level 3.** The learner attaches value to the information and demonstrates a commitment by practicing the newly learned skills. Following the example, on the third visit to this client, the nurse could see that the diet history showed that the client was following his diet creatively by using the new recipes and complying with the diet's restrictions.
- **Level 4.** The learner internalizes the ideas or values. This may be evidenced by extended practice of the new behavior. The client in the example would have, at this point, integrated the new behavior into his or her life-style and be found to have learned this information completely. The client not only understood the special diet but was able to suggest healthy eating strategies for others. The goal of the nurse's care plan in this example had been reached since there was a clear change in the behavior of the client based on a change in values or attitude toward this special diet.

The third and final domain as described by Bloom (1969), is the **psychomotor domain**. The psychomotor domain includes visible, demonstrable performance of skills that require some kind of neuromuscular function. Home care nurses are almost always involved in teaching clients and their families in this domain. The home care nurse's sole responsibility could be to teach a family how to administer insulin to a newly diagnosed diabetic client, a goal specific to the psychomotor domain. Three conditions must be met before psychomotor learning can take place.

1. The learner must have the necessary ability.
2. The learner must have a sensory image of how to carry out the skill.
3. There must be opportunity for practice (Spradley, 1985).

To illustrate these conditions, consider a situation in which a new amputee needs to learn the process of crutch walking. In order for the amputee to be able to crutch walk, he or she must have the necessary ability. This means that there must be one intact leg and a fair amount of upper body strength. This client must also have a mental picture of what crutch walking looks like and how the skill is performed. Once the client knows how to perform the skill, there must be the opportunity to practice crutch walking with the home care nurse or therapist in order for psychomotor learning to take place.

Clearly, cognitive, affective and psychomotor learning are not mutually exclusive. It is almost impossible to teach a client or family about wound care (psychomotor domain) without discussing the concepts of asepsis (cognitive domain) and influencing their values and attitudes about cleanliness (affective domain). So, how does the home care nurse determine which domains pertain to each client situation and develop the teaching plan? This can be done only by applying the concepts of assessment, planning, implementation, and evaluation to the client and family situation. For effective client teaching to occur, the home care nurse must assess the needs of the client and family in each domain and structure her teaching to meet the identified needs.

Assessment

Just as in the nursing process, the first step in the teaching process involves assessment. Assessment of both the learner's readiness to learn and the nurse's ability to teach must be included in this step of the process. The assessment phase of the teaching–learning process provides the foundation for all the steps that follow. Without adequate and accurate data from the assessment, the decisions made and the steps to follow in the remainder of the process will, most likely, be confusing and unproductive for both the nurse and the client.

Assessment of the Learner. The most significant portion of the assessment phase of the teaching–learning process involves assessment of the client's and family's readiness to learn. Many factors affect the client's readiness to learn. These factors include the client's

1. Perceived needs
2. Interests and concerns
3. Educational background
4. Maturational level and age
5. Degree of motivation
6. Cultural, social, religious and economic factors

For example, a client living below the poverty level might be unwilling to learn a new procedure for the care of peripheral vascular ulcers because he or she cannot afford to purchase the supplies needed to perform the procedure. The client resists the teaching of the nurse recognizing that his or her economic situation precludes the client from implementing the teaching done by the nurse.

A factor that affects significantly a client's readiness to learn is motivation. The motivation of the learner is the actual desire to learn. There are two types of motivation that affect the learning process in clients. The first type, intrinsic motivation, is derived from values, attitudes, and the perception that there is an unmet need. A client who wants to learn about exercise in order to integrate an exercise program into his or her daily life may be operating from internal

motivation. Perhaps this client has recently become aware of the value of exercise to a healthy life-style. Perhaps this attitude toward the client's own health has recently changed. The motivation for learning comes from within the client, not from an external source.

The second type of motivation is extrinsic motivation, which stems from such outside forces as family pressure, a change in health status, or environmental factors. Following the above example, if this client's desire to learn about an exercise program is the result of an employer's dictum that he or she should get in shape or be fired, this client's motivation to learn would be external. External motivation is very common in health care situations. Often, some health crisis is the impetus for a client's desire to learn. The client who suffers a myocardial infarction is often highly motivated to learn a low-fat diet in the first few weeks after the attack. Once the impact of the crisis becomes less acute, however, the motivation also becomes less significant, and the client's interest can diminish.

Motivation to learn varies with each client, and any motivation to learn is a valid one. If a client has identified a learning need, it will be helpful if the home care nurse can first identify the client's motivation for learning, since reinforcement of that motivation should be integrated into the teaching plan.

Sources of Data. There are many sources of information that can be used to determine the client's readiness to learn. The first and best source for collecting data about the client will be the client. As a result of the initial and subsequent home visits, the nurse will gather information about those factors that have the potential to influence learner readiness. Additional data can be obtained from the client's family and the significant others involved in the care of the client.

Other sources of data that can be useful in determining the client's readiness to learn include the client care record, including the nursing care plan, and the other health care professionals involved in the client's care. If the client received teaching in the hospital, the professionals involved in that teaching may be instrumental in identifying the client's response to previous teaching, as well as the learning resources used.

In addition to identifying the client's readiness to learn, assessment of the learner will involve the determination of the learning needs of the client. Determination of the learning needs can be made using the same sources used to assess the client's readiness to learn. If a client has recently been discharged from the hospital, valuable information regarding the learning needs of the client and the teaching already accomplished can be obtained from the discharge planner or the primary nurse involved with the client in the hospital.

Although the client will often identify his or her learning needs, the nurse must be able to identify existing as well as potential needs not identified by the client. Through the use of an organized approach (whether it is based on the physiological systems or on the work of a specific nursing theorist), the home care nurse is often able to identify knowledge deficits that may indicate the need for the development of a teaching plan. Existing learning needs of clients are often evident through the assessments made on the initial home visit. For example, during the initial health assessment as part of the admission process, the home care nurse might observe that the client is obese. This would be an indication that diet teaching might need to be included in your care plan even though the client has not identified nutrition as a problem.

Potential learning needs are not always evident to the home care nurse. In order to identify potential learning needs in clients, the home care nurse must know the developmental tasks appropriate for the age of the client being seen in the home. If a home care nurse is seeing an elderly man for wound care following surgery and discovers that the client was recently widowed, potential learning needs might be identified as a result of examining the client's ability to deal with this developmental crisis. Although this would not be the primary purpose of the home visit, a teaching plan addressing this potential learning need could be integrated into the plan dealing with wound care.

Assessment of the Teacher. All too often in the teaching–learning process the focus is on the learner and the information to be conveyed. The characteristics of the teacher also play a crucial role in the teaching–learning process. It is important that the home care nurse assess her teaching abilities carefully before effective teaching can take place. There are four areas that the nurse should assess about herself when developing the teaching plan. These are (1) the knowledge of the material to be taught; (2) the ability to assess the cultural, economic, social, and religious factors; (3) the nurse's skill in teaching; and (4) the potential impact of the nurse's value system on the effectiveness of the teaching.

Assessing how much the home care nurse knows about the material to be taught is integral to the teaching–learning process. Clearly, if a nurse knows very little about a specific medication, the amount she can teach her client about the side effects and methods of administration of that medication will be minimal. Once the home care nurse had identified a gap in her own knowledge, she can consult with other professionals or examine the literature to fill in that knowledge deficit.

As previously discussed, there are many factors that influence the client's ability, readiness, and motivation to learn. Some of those factors include the client's cultural, economic, social, and religious backgrounds. The home care nurse must examine carefully her own ability to assess these factors in the client as they relate to the teaching–learning process. Considering the example of medication teaching, the home care nurse must have the skills to assess the client's ability to purchase the prescribed medications before she implements a teaching plan to foster compliance in taking the medication. A client who is financially unable to purchase the medication will be noncompliant regardless of the amount of knowledge that he or she has about the medication.

The home care nurse's skill in teaching must also be considered in the assessment phase. Some nurses come to home care with a great deal of teaching experience, while others are beginners at this type of intervention. The nurse's skill in teaching may influence the teaching strategies used and affect how comfortable she is implementing the teaching plan. In the above example, a home care nurse who is a novice at teaching might feel more comfortable with a highly structured presentation to the client on the medication, its administration, and the side effects, while an experienced teacher might discuss the material with the client using a handout on the medication as a guide.

The last area of assessment of the teacher involves examining how the nurse's value system might affect the teaching to be done. As in all areas of nursing practice, the values of the nurse must be recognized as an important variable in the implementation of a teaching plan with clients. In the example above, the nurse might be teaching a client about a medication that is part of the client's treatment for drug abuse. If the home care nurse does not recognize her own negative feelings for drug abusers, the implementation of her teaching plan could be seriously compromised. Perhaps the client will sense her negative attitude and feel that it reflects a dislike for him or her personally. Perhaps the nurse's negativism will be evident in a lack of enthusiasm for the material being taught. The nurse's inability to assess her own values related to the teaching to be accomplished will certainly affect the teaching–learning process of the client and the nurse.

Following this self-assessment and the assessment of the learner, the home care nurse is ready to move into the second phase of the teaching–learning process, the planning and implementation phase.

Planning

Setting Objectives. Once the home care nurse has completed her self-assessment and the assessment of the client and family, a sound plan for teaching the client can be developed and implemented. Working with the client and family, the home care nurse needs to identify those behaviors to be acquired by the client as a result of the teaching process. These behaviors are called **objectives** or **goals**. In addition to guiding the development of the teaching plan, learning objectives serve other important purposes.

1. They clearly describe to the client what is expected.
2. They provide a means for evaluation.
3. They allow for coordination of various disciplines in the implementation of the teaching plan.
4. They provide a means of organizing client teaching that will facilitate efficient use of time (Jackson & Johnson, 1988).

There are two characteristics that must be considered in the development of the objectives. An objective must be client centered and measurable. Since an objective is a statement of intended outcome rather than a summary of material to be presented, objectives are *always* written in terms of the behaviors the client will accomplish as a result of the teaching; *never* in terms of what the teacher will do to facilitate the learning. Objectives describe the results of teaching rather than the means of achieving those results. For example, a client-centered and measurable objective would be, after completion of the teaching plan about Digoxin administration, the client will record his pulse on a flow sheet every morning before taking his Digoxin. An example of a nurse-centered objective, which is of little use in evaluating the teaching would be: the nurse will teach the client how to take his pulse and why the pulse should be recorded before taking Digoxin. The latter statement does not reflect the desired change in the client's behavior; therefore, the nurse does not have a means to measure whether the teaching was effective.

The most useful objectives are clear and succinct, leaving little room for interpretation and misunderstanding on the part of the reader. Unfortunately, there are many words used that are open to a wide range of interpretation on the part of the reader. For example, what does it mean when the nurse wants a client to know the four basic food groups? Does she want the client just to be able to say that he or she knows the four food groups, or does she want the client to be able to identify a sample 24-hour intake, with selections from each group? Below is a list of action words that are open to few interpretations, and can be used to write objectives.

To write	To compare
To count	To identify
To list	To record
To define	To recite
To administer	To state

Examples of objectives that are client centered and measurable include the following:

A. After completion of the teaching plan about the four food groups, the client will be able to
1. Identify the four food groups
2. List five foods that are part of each group
3. Plan a day's meals integrating the concept of the four food groups

B. After completion of the teaching plan on care of the abdominal wound, the client will
1. Wash hands before beginning the dressing procedure
2. Assemble all necessary equipment before beginning the procedure
3. Remove the old dressing using unsterile gloves
4. Apply the new dressing using the principles of aseptic technique
5. Wash hands following the dressing procedure
6. Accurately record the amount and type of drainage on a flow sheet

The first set of objectives is clearly related to the cognitive domain while the second set of objectives relates more closely to the psychomotor domain of learning.

Developing a Teaching Plan. Following the development of the learning objectives, the home care nurse can develop the teaching plan. The planning phase involves designing a plan for the learning experience designed to meet the objectives that were developed. Designing the plan includes: 1) identifying the material to be covered; 2) determining the sequence of the material; and 3) selecting the teaching methods that will be used to deliver the specified material. This part of the plan should include a list of the tools (e.g., media, pamphlets, tapes) that can be used to enhance the presentation. A written teaching plan will allow for coordination of the teaching with the various disciplines that may be involved.

Relevance of the subject matter to the client is an important factor in the learning process. Learning takes place more readily and is retained longer if the learner feels that the material is immediately useful. If the client has identified a particular learning need, the nurse is challenged with showing how the learning plan will meet that identified need. When there is little or no recognition that a learning need exists, the greater challenge of helping the client see the lack of skill or knowledge as a problem confronts the home care nurse. With this in mind, **clarifying the learning need** becomes the first step of a teaching plan. Once the learning need is clarified, the home care nurse is faced with making the subject matter relevant to the client's needs.

The home care nurse need only examine the objectives developed in the previous phase of the teaching–learning process to identify the material covered in the teaching plan. Material that helps the client achieve the identified objectives is the material that needs to be included in the teaching plan. For example, if the nurse, in consultation with the client, identified an objective involving the client's ability to identify the side effects of a particular medication, the nurse would then need to teach the client about the side effects as part of her teaching plan. Following the example about the client's ability to change an abdominal wound, if the nurse wants the client to be able to remove the old dressing using an unsterile glove, the nurse needs to include information concerning (1) why it is necessary to use an unsterile glove to remove the dressing (2) how to put on an unsterile glove, (3) how to remove the dressing, and (4) how to discard safely the old dressing material. All this information is derived from the one objective related to the client's ability to remove the old abdominal dressing.

Making a teaching plan relevant to the client also involves planning the method(s) used to deliver the material. Among the many different teaching methods that can be used by the home care nurse, the most traditional methods used in the home are lecture and discussion between the nurse and the client and family. Most commonly, the home care nurse combines the two approaches to teaching, allowing for some time when material is presented to the client followed by a two-way exchange between the nurse and the client and family. Although it can be an excellent method of imparting information efficiently, as a single strategy, the lecture is limited because it creates a passive learning environment. Discussion, as a teaching strategy, gives the learner the opportunity to ask questions, make comments, and receive feedback in order to enhance understanding. This active participation moves the learner further into the learning process.

Demonstration, another teaching method often used for teaching psychomotor skills, is most effective when accompanied by explanations of why the procedure is done in a certain way and by discussions to allow the learner to be more active. Demonstration can give the learner a clear sensory image of how a skill should be performed. When using demonstration as a teaching strategy, it is most helpful to dem-

onstrate with the same kind of equipment the client will be using. The client should have ample opportunity to practice the skill being learned with the nurse present to correct the technique whenever necessary and provide constructive criticism and positive feedback.

The use of audiovisual aids make up a third method of teaching. Audiovisual materials can be used in the teaching plan to enhance the material presented by the teacher. Audiovisual material includes pamphlets, booklets, films, flip charts, audio- and videotapes, and demonstration models. These materials are often available through local chapters of health-related agencies in the community, such as the American Red Cross, the American Heart Association, or the American Cancer Society. Before using any audiovisual aid with a client, the home care nurse must review the material to determine its usefulness in the teaching plan and develop a working knowledge of the material in the presentation. Often, home health agencies have a library of audiovisual materials that are quickly accessible to the nurse; the home care nurse should check with her supervisor.

All written material should be reviewed with the client to determine if the client understands the information being presented in the pamphlet or brochure. It is not enough just to hand someone a brochure or booklet and expect them to go over it unassisted. The nurse should take a few minutes and read important areas with the client, highlighting some points by circling or underlining to be sure that the client reads at least *some* of the material.

It is important to remember that the use of audiovisual aids is also dependent upon the client's ability to see, read, or hear. The inability to read may not be readily apparent to the home care nurse but must be assessed before using any written material as part of the teaching plan. In the course of reviewing written materials with clients, the nurse often can determine that the client is having difficulty reading. If the nurse thinks that the client would not be offended by the question, she may ask the client candidly if he or she is having difficulty reading the specified information. If the nurse decides that the client might be offended by the question, she may ask him or her to relate in the client's own words, what the document says. If the client can not perform this task, the nurse can in a nonjudgmental way, substitute another teaching strategy for the one that involves reading. It may be that the client is unable to read or understand the contents of the document, or perhaps the print in the document is too small for the client to see clearly. Any or all of these factors can affect the client's use of a teaching aid in the learning process. Whatever the cause of the difficulty, the nurse should substitute another teaching strategy for this client and document her assessment in the progress notes and on the client care plan.

In summary, when developing the teaching plan, it is important to remember that learning experiences should provide for the maximum involvement of the client and family. Learning will be enhanced with the active participation of the client in the teaching–learning process. Research has shown that an individual remembers 10% of what is read, 20% of what is heard, 30% of what is seen, 50% of what is heard and seen, 80% of what one says, and 90% of what one says and does (Patterson, 1962). As this research shows, the more of the client's senses that are involved in the learning process, the more likely it is that learning will occur.

Implementation

Implementation of the teaching plan is carried out just like other nursing interventions. Following the first step, assessment of the learner and the teacher, and the second, development of objectives and a teaching plan, the prepared home care nurse should implement the teaching plan with the client and the family. The home care nurse must consider certain factors in the implementation phase of the teaching plan. One of the first considerations is to find an environment conducive to learning in which to carry out the teaching plan. In collaboration with the client and family, the home care nurse must select a noise-free setting that contains the equipment necessary to perform the teaching. Unrelated sound or movement from television or other family members in the home will inhibit the learning process by distracting the teacher or learner, or both. If the learner says the television does not bother him or her, the nurse can say that it bothers her and that she would prefer it to be turned off. In this way the nurse has made the most positive environment possible without making the client feel uncomfortable.

It may be helpful for the home care nurse to ask the client where they could go in the home to do the teaching where they would not be distracted by household noise. If access to a sink is important to the nurse's teaching plan, she should let the client know that the teaching needs to take place either in the kitchen or near the bathroom. Since the setting influences all the teaching that takes place, it must be chosen very carefully and be consistent from visit to visit.

In implementing the teaching plan, certain strategies make the teaching process smoother and facilitate learning on the part of the client. These strategies include

1. Approaching the teaching situation with confidence and enthusiasm. This gives the client the message that the nurse has the knowledge to teach something and that what the nurse has to teach is important

2. Taking time in the presentation and allowing for questions, repetition and reinforcement as needed.

3. Providing lots of positive feedback (praise) to the learner throughout the presentation. Rewards are sometimes helpful, although they should be used in limited situations. An example of a reward sometimes used by home care nurses is spending extra time with a client, either taking him or her for a walk or engaging in some other activity which is out of the ordinary for this client

4. Allowing the client to practice the new skill or use the new information without delay. Learning is reinforced through application

5. Avoiding the use of medical jargon in the teaching process. The use of technical terms can be overwhelming to the client. Try to talk in plain language, repeating if necessary

6. Being sensitive to the client's cues during the teaching process. The nurse might have planned to teach about the diabetic diet and foot care during one home visit but the client seemed exhausted after just learning about the diet. In this situation the nurse would modify her timetable for teaching based on the client's ability to learn. Little learning will take place when the client is tired

7. Requesting client input throughout the teaching program, asking the client to share what he or she knows about the subject and how it relates to his or her life-style and current family situation

8. Summarizing teaching frequently, especially just before ending the teaching session

9. Letting the learner know the progress that was made based on the identified objectives

10. Planning for any subsequent teaching sessions that will be needed

Remember, the good teacher uses this outline

- Tell them what you are going to tell them (Introduction)
- Tell them (implementation of the plan)
- Tell them what you told them (summary of points covered)

The above list covers some suggestions that will help the home care nurse develop the art of client teaching. Since teaching is an art, creativity in one's approach to the teaching process enhances teaching effectiveness. For example, a home care nurse may need to motivate a cardiac client to reduce his intake of sodium. One approach would be to tell the client that he has too much sodium in his diet and suggest that he implement a low-sodium diet. A second, more creative approach would be to take a diet history and show the client, using table salt, how much sodium he consumes in a day from all the foods he eats. The second approach is bound to have a greater impact on the client and result in a more motivated learner. Whether the home care nurse is creative in the approach to the teaching plan or in finding new ways to motivate the learner, teaching and learning are facilitated through the use of creative approaches.

In working with clients in the community, the home care nurse often sees those clients with special learning needs, such as low literacy skills, fatigue that affects the ability to learn, or low motivation. In addition, physiological, psychosocial, economic, and educational factors may provide unique challenges to the development of a meaningful and realistic teaching plan. Adult learners, clients with low literacy skills, and the clients who live in poverty are three populations whose specific characteristics influence the teaching–learning process. Specific approaches to these groups will be discussed further.

The Adult Learner. Home care nurses see clients of all ages in the home but most of their clients and the agency's case load will be over 65 years of age. This population has unique characteristics and needs relating to the teaching–learning process. With an understanding of the adult learner, the home care nurse can design and implement a teaching plan that will meet the learning needs of the client.

The teaching of adults is a field of its own called andragogy. The theory of teaching adults is based on four assumptions that differ from the process of teaching children. These assumptions are

1. As people grow older, their concept of self shifts from one of dependency to one of self-direction
2. They possess a wealth of experience that can be drawn upon in situations
3. Developmental milestones become an impetus for learning
4. Orientation to learning shifts from future to present and from subject to problem (Knowles, 1980)

These four assumptions form the basis for the examination of life. The teachable moment for an adult is when the material and skills to be taught are consistent with the developmental tasks of the adult at that point in his life (Stanhope & Lancaster, 1988).

The final characteristic of the adult learner, and the one that affects the teaching plan most directly is that adults pursue learning for mostly pragmatic reasons. They want to learn in order to be able to do something better or do something they could not do before this time. They may also want to gain information in order to make a decision. The major emphasis of the adult learner is definitely on practical, applied knowledge and skills. The teaching plan must be designed to meet those practical needs of the client. For example, in teaching a client about a diabetic diet, the adult learner will be more interested in and retain more information about the food that should be included in his diet and how that relates to his life-style than about the chemical composition of the carbohydrates and fats.

Taking into account their unique characteristics, the adult learner is just as capable of learning new skills and acquiring knowledge as a child. The home care nurse must remember that the degree of illness will play a role in the learning ability of all clients, not only adult learners. Such factors as degree of pain or fear influence a client's ability and willingness to learn. A client preoccupied with pain is not likely to be able to focus his attention on what the nurse is trying to teach. Similarly, a client with a new colostomy must get over the fear of looking at his or her stoma before the nurse can teach him or her to change the colostomy bag.

Taking into account the physiological needs of the client, the home care nurse can design a meaningful and rewarding learning experience for the adult learner. In developing the learning experience, the nurse must assess the previous learning experiences of the adult client. The nurse can use the same methods to assess the previous knowledge and skills of the adult learner that she would use to assess any other client. These assessment strategies are discussed in the previous section, Assessment.

The Client With Low Literacy Skills. Twenty-three million American adults may not be able to comprehend what a health professional is trying to tell them. These are adults who are either illiterate (cannot read or write) or functionally illiterate. One out of every five American adults is considered functionally illiterate, that is they do not have the literacy skills needed to function effectively in today's society. Generally, they have a reading skill below the fifth grade level. Given the huge numbers of people with low literacy skill, the home care nurse can expect to be providing care to many of these clients in her practice (Doak, Doak & Root, 1985).

Since one of the primary roles of the home care nurse is client education, the client with low literacy skills provides some unique challenges. For clients whose reading, writing, listening, and speaking skills are not well developed, traditional methods of client education may not be appropriate. Research has shown that much of the material published for use by health professionals is client education requires at least an eighth grade reading level. Poor readers and people who do not read at all usually do not ask questions to obtain information. They may not have the skills necessary to develop the question, or they may feel embarrassed by a poor vocabulary. Most people with low literacy skills will cope with new situations by agreeing to whatever is asked of them. For example, when asked, "do you understand?", they may reply "yes" even if they do not understand. This will prevent them from having to explain what they didn't understand. These clients also may not have well-developed problem-solving skills and may have difficulty in classifying information into categories. For example, the client with low literacy skills might have difficulty developing a system for taking several different medications during the day (Hussey & Gilliland, 1989).

When teaching clients with low literacy skills, the nurse may need to make changes in the material and the process of the teaching plan in order to help the client in the achievement of the identified objectives. Assessment of the client's literacy skills is the first step in determining the teaching plan to follow. Imagine the frustration on the part of the home care nurse following a teaching plan that was based solely on written pamphlets and instructions to find out that the client was unable to read what was left as a teaching aid. The home care nurse's frustration is only rivaled by the frustration and embarrassment felt by the client.

Determination of the client's literacy skills can be done very informally by reviewing written material with the client. Through subtle questioning about the content of written material, the nurse can determine the client's ability to comprehend the written word. Asking the client to describe the written material, in the client's own words, is helpful in determining if the client is having difficulty reading or understanding the material in the document used as a teaching aid. If the home care nurse has a question regarding the client's skill in reading, a direct question may be indicated. Most clients respond positively to an honest, caring approach and may even be relieved to share this information so that they can feel more comfortable throughout the learning process. If the client is unable to read, part of the intervention might be a referral to a program that could remedy this problem.

The three strategies identified as central to teaching clients with low literacy skills, emphasize client participation and the assisting of clients in the problem-solving process.

The first strategy involves teaching the smallest amount necessary to reach the stated objectives. Most clients want to learn just enough to allow them to perform the necessary skills. Knowledge for the sake of knowledge is not important to clients with low literacy skills and should be omitted from the teaching plan. Once the nurse has identified the material to be included in the teaching program, it should be reexamined for order and amount of information contained. It may be helpful to teach the skill first, when the client is fully attentive, and then go back to provide some information about the skill later in the visit. For example, when teaching wound care, it would be helpful to teach the skill at the beginning of the visit when the client's attention is at its peak and then teach aseptic principles after that.

The second strategy of teaching patients with low literacy skills is making the points as vividly as possible. The home care nurse can improve vividness by making the sentences short and precise, illustrating the spoken word with drawings and examples, organizing the material with headings and groupings and by summarizing important points. For example, it is much clearer to say, "Change your foot dressing every day," than, "The foot dressing needs to be changed every day." It is often helpful to link new information with old to facilitate recall of material. If a new skill can be shown to be similar to a skill the client already can perform satisfactorily, learning is enhanced. For example, in demonstrating a wound dressing, the use of a bulb syringe could be likened to the use of an eye dropper or even a turkey baster.

The third strategy used in teaching clients with low literacy skills involves providing for repeated reviews. As for all clients, periodic reviews allow for the determination of whether information has been retained or whether misunderstandings have developed throughout the teaching process. Pictures that the client can review independently can be helpful in reinforcing material between visits. There may be a family member or significant other willing to reinforce the teaching if he or she is included in the initial teaching with the client. In addition to reinforcing the material learned, continued reinforcement provides opportunities for continued rewards. Encouraging words are essential in facilitating the learning process.

Teaching strategies may need to be altered with this population of clients. Demonstration and psychomotor practice should replace written information. Diaries and records, which are often used to evaluate adherence to the recommended care regime, may be too difficult for the client with low literacy skills to maintain. If a client has difficulty processing sequence information, a calendar may have little meaning and, therefore, will not be useful as an evaluation strategy. The patient with low literacy skills will benefit from restating or demonstrating the learned material frequently to either the nurse or a family member. The client should be asked to describe what has just been learned, in his or her own words, or demonstrate the skill just acquired. Comprehension occurs when a client can restate what has been learned in his or her own words. Frequent repetition of the learned material or demonstrated ability by both the home care nurse and the client improves the client's ability to recall the new material. The more that clients can rehearse and see themselves in real-life situations, the greater the chances for long-term memory.

Because of the magnitude of the literacy problem in the United States, the home care nurse can expect to see many clients with low literacy skills in practice. Although this population presents some challenges to client education, the modification of traditional teaching strategies will result in a more positive teaching–learning episode. These modifications will yield tremendous benefits in the area of client comprehension and, therefore, will increase the possibility of adherence to a recommended care regime on the part of the client.

The Client in Poverty. Low-income families are seen frequently by the home care nurse in practice. Many factors combine to put the poverty-stricken client at risk for numerous health problems. Factors, such as overcrowded living conditions, limited education, and difficulty in using available resources, make the problems of the poverty-stricken seem overwhelming for the family and the home care nurse alike.

Poverty, a relative term, reflects a judgment made on the basis of standards prevailing in the community. For the purpose of this discussion, the client to be addressed is one who lives in a chronic state of poverty, poverty that spans many generations and is an accepted way of life. Due to limited education, this client is often unable to find meaningful or regular work. Feelings of low self-esteem are reinforced by the inability to maintain regular employment.

Clients who live in a chronic state of poverty have four distinctive life themes that tend to characterize their behaviors. These life themes include fatalism, orientation to the present, authoritarianism, and concreteness (Aleman, 1982). All these life themes affect the material and method of teaching to be used by the home care nurse. Consideration of these life themes is essential to making the teaching process meaningful for the client living in a chronic state of poverty.

Fatalism results from a strong feeling of powerlessness. Often, clients have many external forces, such as their case worker, the food stamp program, or the welfare office, controlling their lives. Since they often feel at the mercy of these external forces, they lose all motivation to learn. Recognizing that motivation is a critical element in the teaching–learning process, the home care nurse must help the client find either an internal or external motivation for learning.

The second life theme, orientation to the present, is seen as a result of the client having to spend a great deal of time obtaining satisfiers of such basic needs as food, housing, and fuel. After these tasks are accomplished, little time or energy remain for planning for the future. Since the availability of resources to meet basic needs is not assured, the client becomes preoccupied with the present, unable to plan ahead or delay gratification. For the home care nurse trying to teach this client, the existence of this characteristic provides unique challenges. The benefits of a behavior change that will improve long-term health status are not likely to be valued by the client with an orientation to the present. Furthermore, the client occupied with meeting basic needs may not be interested in the teachings of the home care nurse. Recognition of this life theme is essential in planning the teaching–learning process with poverty-stricken clients.

Authoritarianism is the third life theme often seen in clients in poverty. Decision making in these families is often situational and based on authority. The person in charge makes the decisions for others. The home care nurse must identify the person in charge. Once that person is identified, the home care nurse could enlist that individuals's support and assistance. The home care nurse can increase her credibility and effectiveness by establishing a liaison with the influential people in the client's community.

Concreteness is the final life theme often seen in clients in poverty. In these clients, life is seen to be very concrete and activity oriented. Action is valued, emotions are expressed in visible, tangible ways. Listening tends not to be a reinforced skill. Everyone may talk at once, trying to be the loudest to get the desired attention. This life theme has direct implications for the teaching–learning process. The home care nurse can best meet the learning needs of her clients through an action-oriented teaching plan, with little emphasis on learning through listening. Perhaps demonstration could replace oral instructions for this client to meet most effectively the specified learning need. This client should be actively, tangibly involved in each step of the teaching–learning process.

These four life themes combine to make teaching clients in poverty a challenge for the home care nurse. With some extra planning and an innovative approach to interventions, teaching can be effective and rewarding.

Evaluation

Just as it is in the nursing process, evaluation is the final step in the teaching-learning process. Although this step is critical to determining the success of the teaching, it is often forgotten or ignored. There are two areas that can be addressed in evaluation of the teaching–learning process; evaluation of the teaching effectiveness and evaluation of the teacher performance.

Evaluation of the teaching effectiveness can be done by examination of the objectives that were developed at the beginning of the process. The objectives were statements of the anticipated client behaviors that should be present at the conclusion of the teaching. As the home care nurse examines the identified objectives, a determination of whether the client met the objective can be made. Determination of what the client learned can be made by return demonstrations, written tests, documentation of the client's behaviors in progress notes and examination of self-reported information, such as diaries and logs. Although all these methods are useful, the most frequent evaluative measure used by the home care nurse is oral questioning of the client. The home care nurse will often say "Tell me what you had for breakfast this morning, and lunch and supper yesterday" to determine the effectiveness of the diet teaching that was performed. If the client has met the objective, the teaching plan can be considered successful.

If the objective was not accomplished, there are several areas to examine to determine why the stated objectives were not met.

1. Perhaps the objectives were unrealistic or too complex for the client to meet in the time available.
2. If it is impossible to determine if the learner has met the objectives, the learning objectives may not be client centered or measurable.
3. The teaching strategy may not have been appropriate for the learning objective. For example, if the objective called for the client to learn a new skill and the teaching method was exclusively the lecture, the teaching strategy was not appropriate for the learning objective.
4. Perhaps the learner was not motivated to learn what was included in the teaching plan.

This points to the need for inclusion of the learner at each step of the process, including the development of the objectives. The home care nurse should also determine if the instructional aids were useful and suitable. If it was determined that the teaching was unsuccessful or incomplete for any reason, the entire process begins again, starting with assessment.

Evaluation of the performance of the teacher is important for both the client and the professional development of the home care nurse. The home care nurse may simply want to ask the client for feedback on her effectiveness as a teacher. Peers and supervisors may be asked to review the teaching plan on the client record to provide insight on the home care nurse's strengths and weaknesses as a teacher. If an in-depth evaluation is needed, a supervisor or peer can make a joint visit with the home care nurse to assess the teaching more thoroughly. Most likely, most information about the effectiveness of the teacher will be obtained through self-evaluation on the part of the home care nurse. Following implementation of the teaching plan, the home care nurse may reflect on her familiarity with the subject taught and the degrees of confidence, openness, and mutual respect that were displayed to the client. All these factors will have an impact on the degree of success of the teaching–learning process for both the client and the home care nurse.

The evaluation phase may end the nurse–client relationship or it may lead to the identification of further problems to be addressed. It can never be assumed that because teaching was done, learning has taken place. Evaluation *must* be done as the final phase of the teaching–learning process.

Client Compliance. *Webster's New Collegiate Dictionary* defines compliance as "the act or process of complying to a desire, demand, or proposal or to coercion." As professionals, home care nurses hardly want to think of their role as involving coercion. Although nurses want their clients to adhere to their recommended care regime, that adherence ideally, should come as a result of an understanding by the client that certain behaviors are more beneficial to his or her health status than others. As a result of a therapeutic relationship in which health teaching is conducted, the client should gain the necessary knowledge and skills to make wise choices about his or her health based on the developed care regime.

Client compliance is a complex behavior that is affected by many variables. A key factor in achieving client compliance is the nurse's relationship with the client, including a respect for the client's values, individuality, and autonomy. The client must be viewed as a partner in the teaching process rather than as a passive recipient of information (Leff, 1986). Compliance increases if the client and nurse share their concerns and goals for care.

A second factor that influences compliance is a clear understanding by the client of the relationship between the prescribed care regime and the prevention or treatment of illness. Once that relationship has been established, the nurse is often charged with helping the client to see the importance of the desired change in relation to the client's short- or long-term health status. This is a necessary and often difficult step on the road to compliance, especially when the changes involve behaviors that have been long standing. Contracts between the nurse and the client may be helpful in this process since the client can clearly identify the desired behaviors. Contracting is discussed in detail earlier in this chapter.

Research has not shown a clear relationship between knowledge and compliance. In other words, there is no assurance that a client will comply with a prescribed diet just because he or she has the necessary information to plan a healthy meal appropriately. Recognizing this limitation, certain techniques or strategies can be used to increase compliance. These strategies include

- Simplification of care regime. The home care nurse should always begin with the simplest activities and build to more complex actions. Also, any activities included to reduce the overall complexity of the client situation will enhance compliance.
- Allowing change to occur slowly. Compliance will be improved if the client is allowed to make changes in his or her life slowly. This allows the client to adapt his or her life-style to the prescribed change without major disruption.
- Enlisting family support. A client's likelihood of compliance is increased if the family is supportive of the change. Family support is often necessary since a behavior change in the client may affect the family members.
- Increased client supervision. Increased supervision of clients can be accomplished by scheduling more frequent home visits for follow-up and practice of the skills or by enlisting the caregivers' help in working more closely with the client. Increasing the frequency of home visits must always be done with consideration for the reimbursement potential for the visit.

Recognizing that client compliance is not always associated with increased education, the home care nurse must consider the above listed strategies in order to enhance the potential for compliance. It must be stressed that the first and most significant variable in promoting compliance is a therapeutic relationship between a nurse and client in which the client plays an active role in the decision making and the goal setting with regard to the plan of care.

Potential Problems in Teaching. Client teaching, like other areas of nursing practice, does not always go as smoothly as the home care nurse would hope. There are often unforeseen circumstances that affect the client's receptivity to the teaching plan or the nurse's ability to deliver effectively the anticipated intervention. The nurse can learn from her mistakes. Although difficulty in teaching may be encountered at any point in the teaching–learning process, common potential problem areas will be identified, and strategies to deal with these problems will be discussed.

Goals are established by mutual agreement between the client and the nurse. **Failure to negotiate goals** can lead to the nurse and client working toward different and often conflicting ends. Goals are a dynamic part of the teaching–learning process, that is, they need to change as the client situation changes. Periodic renegotiation of goals between the client and the home care nurse is essential.

The specific characteristics of the client are important in the teaching–learning process. It must be remembered that the nurse is sometimes teaching a client with a reduced attention span and endurance due to some past or present illness. Sometimes the patient will be in pain or distracted by fatigue or anxiety. **Patient overload** will result from presenting too much material in too short a time. If possible, shorter sessions occurring more frequently will help to avoid this problem.

Sequencing of the activities in the visit must also be considered. Often difficulties that relate to the **poor timing of client teaching** arise in the teaching process. For example, if a home visit involved a complicated wound dressing and a teaching session, it might be better to perform the teaching first, before the client becomes distracted with the wound care.

Audiovisual aids can be an asset to the home care nurse in the planning and delivery of client education. **Poor use of audiovisual aids** does little to facilitate learning and may even impede the learning process. The home care nurse must always review the material before using it with a client. Important points in the media should be stressed or highlighted for the client. Never rely solely on an audiovisual aid to perform the teaching. Aids should be used to supplement or enhance the nurse's presentation, not as a substitute for teaching.

Failure to validate all areas of client information is the final potential problem area to be discussed. When the nurse makes assumptions about a client's motivation, previous knowledge, or level of understanding about the client's illness, she will be basing important decisions on information that may be false. This can lead to an inefficient use of the nurse's time and a frustrating learning experience for the client. The best way to find out what the client knows about his or her illness is to ask. In every step of the teaching–learning process, assessment, planning, intervention, and evaluation, the nurse must validate all information about the client with the client. In this way, the nurse can be sure that her decision is based on accurate information.

Although not an exhaustive list, these few potential problem areas are seen frequently in the home care setting. The home care nurse should consider these areas when devising and implementing a teaching plan for her client.

Documentation

Following the implementation and evaluation of the teaching plan, the home care nurse must carefully and thoroughly document each stage of the teaching plan. The need for documentation of client teaching for the purpose of continuity of care and as part of the nurse's responsibility as a health care professional is readily apparent. Assessment of the client's knowledge deficit and documentation of client teaching are both crucial elements in determining the reimbursement of the home visit through third party payors, such as Medicare. Documentation of a carefully outlined teaching plan, description of the teaching to be done, and the client's and family's responses to that teaching is necessary to demonstrate that the teaching that was done was indeed reimbursable.

In attempting to help clients reach the goal of independence, client education is one of the most frequent interventions used by home care nurses. Although used often as part of the care plan, client education is frequently undocumented or under-documented by the practitioner. It is suggested that

> Teaching is probably one of the most under-documented skilled services because most nurses in home care do not recognize the scope and depth of the teaching they do. The teaching is often done in an informal, conversational, and sometimes reactive manner. Nurses tend to view much of their teaching as common-sense suggestions. Yet, such suggestions are based on the nurse's professional education and experience (Omdahl, 1987, pg. 1033).

In order to document effectively the process of client teaching, the home care nurse must first know what constitutes a skilled teaching visit. Under the Medicare program, specific criteria have been established that determine whether a teaching visit is reimbursable. In general, home health benefits under Medicare are reimbursable for intermittent skilled services for a client in the acute or subacute phases of an illness. Chronic care, even when it is skilled, is not considered reimbursable by Medicare. Given this general criterion, several factors can be used to determine if teaching visits are reimbursable under the Medicare program.

One criterion used by Medicare to determine if the teaching visit is reimbursable is examination of the person who conducted the teaching. Skilled care, which requires professional health training, is performed by registered or licensed nurses and therapists. Teaching that requires the expertise of one of these health care professionals is considered reimburs-

able under the Medicare program. When the nature of the service is such that it can be performed adequately by a person without professional training, that service is not reimbursable regardless of who performs it. For example, if the home care nurse taught a client about a diabetic diet, that teaching would be reimbursable because it required the professional training of the nurse to accomplish. On the other hand, if the professional nurse told a client with edema to elevate his or her feet, that would not be considered skilled care because most nonmedical people have enough knowledge to do this in the event of swelling (Jackson & Johnson, 1988).

It also must be remembered that the teaching of a skill to a client or family member, as well as the performance of that skill, may be considered reimbursable. When a home care nurse teaches a family member a skill, after the skill is mastered, the family member functions as the skilled provider. A situation in which the family member becomes unable to perform that skill for the client, performance of the procedure will be considered a skilled service if performed by the nurse (Jackson & Johnson, 1988).

The second criterion used to determine if the teaching visits are reimbursable by Medicare is the reasonableness and necessity of the teaching that is done. To be considered **reasonable** and **necessary** for the treatment of an illness or injury, the services must be consistent with the nature and severity of the individual's illness and injury, his particular medical needs, and the accepted standard of practice for clients with like conditions (Medicare, April 1989, sec 204.3). Examination of the nature and severity of the illness is the first stage in determining the amount of teaching to be done. For example, a client who has been a diabetic, administering insulin for 20 years would not require an extensive teaching plan about insulin administration unless it could be determined and documented by the nurse that severe knowledge deficits and misunderstandings were present.

The home care nurse must be especially careful with the reinforcement of teaching to clients. As mentioned, reinforcement is a necessary part of the teaching–learning process. For reinforcement, fewer visits would be needed than for initial training. Repeated teaching is generally not reimbursable unless changes which justify the intervention are noted by the nurse. For example if a 2g sodium diet was taught to a cardiac client and the physician changed the diet order to a 1g sodium diet, reinforcement of a low-sodium diet would be indicated. When documenting client teaching, the nurse should try to avoid using such words as reinforced, reviewed, or reminded. Whenever possible, link reinforcement of previous teaching with documentation about new teaching that was performed. Remember, Medicare may reimburse for one visit to reinforce teaching, but reimbursement would not extend further.

Client compliance with the new information learned is another factor in determining whether teaching visits are reimbursable. The purpose of the teaching–learning process is to help the client improve function and manage disease. If the home care nurse determines that the client continues to be unable to manage his or her disease following implementation of the teaching plan, a determination must be made for the reason of the lack of compliance. Evaluation of the teaching plan will help determine if the teaching strategies used were inappropriate and thereby blocked learning. In some cases, the client will achieve the desired objectives if more time than originally allotted is provided. If the client will not comply with instructions even though learning has been determined to have taken place, further teaching visits would not be reimbursable. Periodic reevaluation of the client's progress toward a specified learning objective is essential to the reimbursement process.

Considering all the factors that are evaluated to determine if a service is reimbursable under the Medicare program, the home care nurse must document all assessment and teaching clearly and as specifically as possible. One of the major flaws in documenting teaching is that the home care nurse writes about teaching in general terms. In order to facilitate clarity of documentation, the home care nurse must ask, "Why am I telling the client this?" and "What impact should this teaching have on this patient?" (Omdahl, 1987). In order to make the documentation clear and specific. therefore increasing the likelihood of reimbursement for the teaching visit, the following items can be included in the client record.

1. Date and time of the teaching session
2. To whom the teaching is directed; if not the client, why?
3. Client's health status
4. Specific instructions given
5. Teaching method used
6. Patient's level of comprehension
7. Barriers to the teaching process
8. Goals that were met during the teaching session
9. Evaluation of the teaching session
10. Plans for the next teaching session (Jackson and Johnson, 1988, p. 64)

Inclusion of all these items in the written narrative notes may result in a rather lengthy submission, but it is all material that needs to be included to justify Medicare services. Some agencies use flow sheets or checklists to facilitate quick, yet complete charting. A flow sheet may be adequate for recording basic information regarding the teaching episode, but the nurse must realize that a flow sheet can and should be supplemented with narrative charting as the need arises. If all the above items can be included on the flow sheet, no narrative charting is needed. If not, a narrative note to supplement those areas not addressed on the flow sheet is indicated. Figure 4–1 is an example of a teaching flow sheet. The home care nurse should discuss the use of flow sheets with the nursing supervisor.

Home care nurses need to recognize the important role that client education plays in their practice. An understanding of the process of client education and the method chosen to document that process is crucial to a positive educational outcome for the client and reimbursement for the agency.

TEST YOURSELF

1. What model of home care nursing delivery do you use in your agency? How does that affect the way you practice?

2. What tools are available in your agency to assist you in case load management?

3. How does your agency assure that clients don't "fall through the cracks" and that visits are not missed?

Problem/knowledge deficit		Objectives/goals				
		Upon completion of the teaching, the client will				
1.		a.				
2.		b.				
3.		c.				
4.		d.				
5.		e.				

Date						
Time						
Who was taught						
Response to teaching						
Teaching intervention / Goals met						
a.						
b.						
c.						
d.						
e.						
f.						

CODE
P: Instructions provided, learning progressing, continues to need teaching
C: Instructions provided, teaching completed
N: Instructions provided, noncompliant

Signature/Title

Figure 4–1. Teaching flow sheet

4. List five time-wasters and five time-savers you can anticipate will affect your practice. Think about these time-wasters and time-savers again 3 and 6 months after your initial employment date.

5. What client assessment information determined on a home visit indicates that you should plan a visit for the next day?

6. Case example: Mr. Jones is a 60-year-old man who was discharged yesterday from the hospital following an aortic valve replacement. Surgery and the postoperative course were uneventful except for two periods of arrythmia that occurred 1 day before discharge. Mr. Jones was referred to home care for diet teaching and assessment of his cardiac status. Before surgery, Mr. Jones was a long-distance truck driver for a major moving company. He plans to return to this job as soon as his doctor permits, since he is only 3 years from retirement. Since Mr. Jones spends weeks away from home, he eats many of his meals at fast-food restaurants and diners. He feels that this way of life is inevitable, given his job and its requirements.

   Mr. Jones has been married for 35 years and has two grown children who live out of the house. His wife would like to see him change his eating habits but is unwilling to confront him on this subject because she sees him as "the boss."

   Based on this example

   a. What things would you need to consider before setting up a contract with Mr. Jones?

b. Describe the main points you would discuss with Mr. Jones about contracting.

c. Outline the contract you would develop with Mr. Jones.

7. What problems do you think you will find in contracts with clients and their families?

8. Mrs. Brown is a frail 76-year-old woman who lives with her 68-year-old, unmarried sister. Both are retired school teachers and are able to live comfortably on their pensions and social security. Mrs. Brown was discharged from the hospital following a 2-week stay for treatment of a peripheral vascular ulcer. Before her hospitalization, Mrs. Brown bumped her leg on her bedpost. At first, the bump resulted in a 1-inch abrasion. The wound opened and started weeping, and Mrs. Brown treated herself with baking soda compresses and Tylenol. By the time she saw her doctor, the wound was 3 inches around and ½ inch deep with purulent yellow drainage. She also had a fever of 101.6 F. Mrs. Brown is diabetic and is treated with oral hypoglycemic agents.
Mrs. Brown was referred for home care services for wound care to the partially healed ulcer. Since the client is diabetic, the doctor feels that the healing time will be prolonged, with total time of approximately 3 months. Orders for home care include teaching the client and caregiver the wound care procedure.
a. What are the main issues that need to be addressed as part of the initial assessment for Mrs. Brown?

b. Identify three objectives or goals for this teaching plan.

c. Develop a teaching plan in order to accomplish the wound care instruction.

d. What unique characteristics of this client situation must be taken into consideration in implementing the teaching plan?

e. Think about a teaching session that could take place with this client, and document all significant elements of the session.

9. What are the strategies you can use to make the teaching–learning experiences positive for both the client and yourself?

10. What techniques have you found successful in teaching clients who are labeled "noncompliant"?

Interpersonal Aspects of Home Care Nursing

OBJECTIVES

Upon completion of this chapter the reader will be able to identify
1. The purposes of supervision
2. A definition of supervision
3. Expectations of supervision from the perspective of both the staff nurse and the supervisor
4. The roles and functions of the supervisor
5. The role of the home care nurse as supervisor of paraprofessionals
6. The three leading causes of stress in home care nurses
7. Ways in which the home care nurse can manage stress

KEY CONCEPTS

- **Definition of supervision**

- **Key supervisory roles**

- **Supervisor as orientation coordinator**

- **How to supervise a home health aide**

- **Ways for the home care nurse to manage stress**

AGENCY-SPECIFIC MATERIALS NEEDED:

- Organizational Chart
- Mission and philosophy of organization
- Home health aide activity sheet
- Home health aide policies relating to visits and RN supervision
- Documentation record for orientation and supervision of home health aide
- Productivity standards and ways of evaluating productivity
- Professional reference material available (e.g., books, journals)
- Nurse personnel evaluation schedule and policies
- Schedule and policies of in-service and continuing education

INTRODUCTION

The field of home care nursing can be professionally challenging for the nurse, especially working with clients and families in the home and community. The home care nurse must understand that her relationship with her clients is important, but that there are also interpersonal aspects of the job that require equal attention. Being supervised and supervising the work of others is an important component of the home care nurse's role, especially since this type of practice is so independent, yet interdependent. Additionally, if the nurse is not aware of the work stressors unique to home care nursing she is likely to experience burnout and frustration that can have an impact on her personal as well as professional life. This chapter covers the two major interpersonal aspects of home care nursing—supervision in home care and stress. Discussion of the issues as well as guidelines and exercises included in this chapter can help the nurse to succeed in these two important areas.

SUPERVISION IN HOME CARE

Successful performance of staff nurse functions in a home care agency depends on philosophical harmony with the mission of the agency and the beliefs of all the staff. Most agencies have a mission statement that guides organizational planning and purpose. It is not enough to believe that staff supervision is a mutual educational and administrative effort. This belief must be demonstrated through practice in professional relationships. The staff nurse is the agency's primary representative to the community and conveys the agency message of its mission and standards of care by the way nursing in the home is practiced. It is the staff nurse who brings life to the agency's goals and mission.

The method by which the nurse relates and carries out the clinical work through practice is a dynamic process and, as with any experience, maturing in the role does much to enhance success. Bringing together the primary roles of staff development and administrative management skills is the function and process of supervision that guides and directs nursing practice. The staff nurse has the most contact with and is most influenced and affected by the supervisor. Early in a staff nurse's experience, a discussion about the purpose and expectations of supervision is very important.

The Purposes of Supervision

The first purpose of supervision is to facilitate and accomplish work through the staff worker. This involves carefully planned and timely participatory exchanges between the staff nurse and the supervisor. Communication should be candid and, at times, critical with emphasis placed on how the supervisor can help make the staff member's work more successful.

A second purpose of supervision is to see that the care rendered by the staff nurse or other worker, to the client and the family, is safe and appropriate. Concern for public safety is of prime importance for both the home care nurse and the supervisor. Should there be any evidence of a threat to safe nursing practice, the supervisor must immediately take steps to see that it is corrected. Corrective steps include counseling, observing the care as it is being given, and being certain that the needed educational opportunities are made available for the nurse.

A third purpose of supervision is to facilitate staff development. This should include both an individualized plan and an agency commitment to guide the staff member toward improved clinical practice and build for greater growth in the nursing profession. Facilitating staff is important, but all too often it is not seen as requiring major effort. Developing leadership from within the staff ranks is important, but many supervisors may not have a planned approach for achieving this goal with staff members. The supervisor and staff member should discuss goals as an integral part of the relationship between them and lay out a plan for progressive experience based on demonstrated success in earlier work. Developing staff can lead to the staff nurse's growth in more responsible positions within the organization. Supervisors of talented staff nurses will want to reap the benefits of work done. It is right for the supervisor to take pride in observing a staff worker making progress and contributing to the profession, regardless of whether the nurse stays with the home care agency or moves to another work situation.

Defining Supervision

The word *supervision* brings to the minds of many an image of an overbearing, order-giving, authority, demanding certain behavior and acting as a "checker-upper" on the work of the staff member. While it is hard for the supervisor to avoid some of that description, for the staff nurse, supervision can be positive, feeling good about the work done and knowing that advice is available if and when it is needed, not only having one's work scrutinized. Unfortunately, supervision is often thought about in negative rather than in positive terms.

One definition of supervision that should be primary to the home care nurse is that of an enabling person through which staff workers are helped to make the best use of their knowledge or skills, to improve them, and to do the job better. Supervision should be viewed as emphasizing the helping and nurturing aspect of relationships. The ultimate goal is to fulfill the agency's mission through more effective efforts on the part of its workers. The supervisor is the person in the middle who represents the agency and its administration to the staff workers and the workers to the administration.

Expectations

Growth and development in clinical practice as a staff nurse parallel some of the stages used to describe human development. Many changes can take place within each stage, but a person moves from one to the next as new skills and tasks are accomplished and builds toward increasingly more difficult skills and more defined use of clinical judgment. Therefore, the pace of clinical practice expertise is not the same for each nurse. Accordingly, each has needs and expectations that require individual planning and implementation.

Expectations of the Staff. New staff nurses will expect the supervisor to explain and describe the background of the agency and the role and tradition it has filled in the community over the years it has been in business. They will need specific instruction about techniques, procedures, community resources, case load management, time management, and organizational skills. A staff nurse will want the supervisor to explain the appropriate channels of communication and to provide information on how and why a policy or procedure was developed.

An experienced staff member will want freedom to develop ideas, to be creative, and to take on increasing independence. Further, the nurse should expect opportunities to broaden her clinical practice and look to the supervisor for ways to achieve this. Finally, a home care nurse will expect assistance in expanding clinical competence and to have a good measure of job satisfaction as a result.

The supervisor is a role model for the staff nurse who focuses clinical decision-making skills that are basic to competent staff nurse home care practice. The staff nurse should be encouraged to begin to buy selected reference books and subscribe to journals that will enhance her base of clinical knowledge.

Expectations of the Supervisor. An expectation of the supervisor is to have a positive influence on the quality of home care services provided by the agency and to provide leadership that results in efficiency and job satisfaction for the staff member. Of course, the supervisor is influenced by previous work experiences and by the size and scope of the agency's services. Again, expectations are shaped by what the supervisor feels comfortable and competent doing. New and unfamiliar aspects of supervision require more concentration and time to develop a level of confidence.

The nurse's supervisor wants her to feel free to seek and to accept direction in new experiences and to have the support of the agency to guide and foster competence in the role. A constant flow of new information must be assimilated and used in caring for the home care client. It is the supervisor who is most likely to make this information available to staff nurses. The agency will purchase books and reference materials, subscribe to special resources, and find ways to facilitate the use of other provider specialists so that pertinent clinical information is made available for staff. Even as the staff nurse begins building a clinical library, the supervisor, too, expands subscription lists during this time and builds a personal professional library that can be shared with staff.

Expectations of the Administrator. The administrator is usually involved in the outside affairs of the home care agency, while the supervisor and staff nurse are focused on the day-to-day activities. In the same way that supervisors get their work done through staff members, administrators get a measure of their work done through the supervisor. Administrators will expect the staff to be knowledgeable and continue to learn abut the role of the agency, the scope of safe clinical practice in the home and to some extent, the larger health care system. The administrator expects the work unit to be managed effectively and to be efficient in providing services and enhancing staff productivity. Whenever it is necessary, interpretation of agency policy and services to others in the community is expected to be done at times by the supervisor or staff nurse. It is an integral part of the staff role to offer to participate in clinical development of peers as a role model and to demonstrate team work among colleagues. The administrator expects support and loyalty from both supervisors and staff nurses as well as a partnership in providing the best home care available.

Balancing Supervisory Roles and Functions

The home care nurse must become acquainted with the breadth and functions of the supervisory roles. There are many responsibilities that fall to the supervisor and that are not often recognized by staff nurses as being essential. These responsibilities can be divided into three categories: administrative, educational/staff development, and communications linkages. The staff nurse is the primary beneficiary of all of these. It is possible to identify certain duties for each category that will highlight the broad practice scope of the nursing supervisor in a home care agency.

Some of the supervisor's administrative duties include

- Managing the work flow of all workers in a designated unit
- Participating in planning, development, and evaluation of agency programs
- Participating in planning, development, and evaluation of agency policies that affect the delivery of home care services
- Hiring and terminating professional staff
- Managing the quality assurance program for the work unit
- Assisting in the budget process for the work unit
- Collecting and analyzing service, statistical and fiscal data
- Monitoring the worker's productivity and fiscal activities of the work unit
- Facilitating and participating in research activities

Selected educational and staff development responsibilities include

- Helping staff members, individually and as a group, to learn and to build on that learning as an orientation experience or later on, as an experienced staff nurse
- Developing and implementing recording formats so that necessary and current information is provided for more informed clinical practice
- Encouraging and facilitating staff participation in agency and professional activities
- Preparing formal and informal performance evaluations to aid in growth of staff members
- Fostering formal and informal educational efforts and facilitating staff participation in continuing education, in-service education, and academic education programs

Some functions in enhancing communications include

- Providing a forum for open communication between upper level management and staff nurses
- Representing the agency in the community in formal and informal ways
- Collaborating with other home care providers in planning and providing services to the ill at home
- Informing staff about regulatory changes or policies that influence the home care services being provided

These lists highlight the scope of responsibilities that a clinical supervisor has in a home care agency. While the staff nurse is the direct recipient of the performance of these duties, all who relate with the home care agency benefit from them. The staff nurse and the supervisor work so closely together that it goes unnoticed that the supervisor influences so many aspects of the home care agency service. By understanding the supervisor's activities the staff nurse becomes a potential supervisor.

Limits of Supervision

There are limitations to what can be provided by the supervisor. Identifying the boundaries of supervisory practice is essential; it is easy for the nurse to expect too much from her supervisor and then be disappointed when the expectations are not met.

One limitation is that the supervisor and the nurse do not work in the same setting. The supervisor cannot be present at every move and action of the staff nurse. This is especially true in home care where the clinical activities are performed in a home without other advisors available except by telephone. The supervisor should function much like a coach on a playing field. The coach does not play a position or cover a base but expects the player to do that. Similarly, in home care the work is delegated to the staff nurse, and it is expected that the care will be done appropriately following instructions.

Another aspect of supervision that may be viewed as a limitation, is that while the relationship between staff and supervisor is close, it should be an independent relationship. The supervisor should not be seen as a counselor for personal problems, although it may be necessary for the supervisor to advise and refer a worker for assistance if outside problems interfere with work.

Key Supervisory Roles

Orientation. When a new staff nurse begins work at a home care agency, it is the supervisor who arranges for and provides a large part of the orientation that is necessary for learning the work. This is one of the most important functions of the supervisor, next to the ongoing day-to-day clinical supervision that is in place for staff. The initial orientation includes basic information concerning the client care record, selected agency client care policies and procedures and other information provided in this book. Spending a day with other nurses acquaints the new nurse with the typical visiting day and associated activities.

As was discussed in chapter 1, discussion about the philosophy and mission of the agency should be included in orientation so that the new nurse can begin to think and "feel" what that means in practice. This should be reviewed during a job interview, but it becomes relevant during the orientation period when the nurse puts it into practice. Orientation is intense and while the new nurse may not be out making visits and working hard in caring for a client in the home, the nurse will be tired and fatigued by the end of the day because of all the information that must be remembered.

After this initial time of learning about home care, the agency, and some of the usual activities, the orientation moves toward more clinical work. For instance, the scope of home care nursing practice begins to help the nurse think about and do some case load management, then she is introduced to community resources and related content. This is one of the most important times in any staff worker's life, and it is also one of the most difficult times because it seems so distant from the real work. Home care, for some, is medical–surgical nursing moved from the hospital to the home. Although home care nursing can include medical–surgical work, the scope is much broader because family and community are important aspects to include in a plan of care, as discussed in chapter 2.

Staff Motivation. Often one hears administrators or supervisors say that a certain staff member "is such a pleasure" to have on the agency staff. Just what is it that makes that person so special? When it comes down to it, often it is that the nurse is highly motivated and excited about the work, shows initiative, and finds professional and intellectual stimulation through supervisory contact. This can be a problem for the supervisor who has many people to supervise with not all staff members equally motivated in their work. The staff member, resistant and demonstrating little or no individual initiative, is difficult, but not impossible, to deal with. Such people can cause particular problems if they complain frequently and influence other staff members in the work unit by using a divide and conquer tactic. Studies have identified some common factors that predict an increase in motivation on the job. These include a sense of achievement, recognition, and responsibility, with salary near the end of a list of eight items. The use of tangible rewards, usually money, is one way to recognize and motivate a staff worker. Placing too high a value on money can be risky since, in some ways, money is the easiest reward to give but it may be offered at the expense of other rewards that do more to promote professional growth. Other ways a staff member can be rewarded would be attendance or participation at a professional conference, subscription to a professional journal of choice, or the purchase of a clinically appropriate book.

Productivity. Productivity is a reflection of motivation, and if staff workers feel a sense of "ownership" of their product (clinical service), they will show a measurable level of achievement.

Productivity is viewed by some as one type of management control. Measuring actual output or work done by staff and comparing it with budgeted expectations is increasingly common in home care agencies, and it can influence the revenue that can be assigned to support staff activities including staff salaries. This may be viewed by staff as a punishing approach, but the fact is that when chargeable visits are made and accounted for, there is a direct impact on the income side of the agency ledger. The escalating cost of health care, including home care, is a total agency concern, not just one for the board of directors and the administrators. Improving the efficiency of staff workers is an essential part of the productivity strategy. There may well be ways that the staff nurse can focus on the clinical assessment and intervention of a home visit and not have to attend to the many other important details pertaining to admission and billing. Perhaps a time has been reached when a nonclinical person can complete these parts of the information beginning with securing data by phone and possibly a follow-up home visit. Hospitals have nonclinical staff handling the admissions process, and many home care agencies are considering the same thing. This reduces the burden on the staff nurse of nonclinical work with the result of greater productivity in substance and numbers of home visits to clients. Staff workers, especially nurses, have much material to keep in mind when recording a visit. There are many details, mostly appropriate, to put onto the clinical record and onto various forms that must be submitted for accounting purposes. Agency administrators can come up with a variety of system changes to facilitate the nurses' work, but the effective use of these systems depends on the nurse. All of this work is necessary as a part of demonstrating productivity levels. This responsibility is shared by the supervisor and the staff worker.

Staff Development. Development activities with the new employee initially will focus on proficiency in the day-to-day work. As the staff nurse gains experience, efforts can be directed towards other issues involving home care. In the beginning of a staff nurse's work experience, the supervisor should establish a system of regular conferences for the purposes of coaching and planning case load management. Aside from working with an individual staff nurse toward early independence in clinical practice, staff development is aimed at increasing the clinical competence of a staff group. Staff development is a process rather than a structured program and, as such, it is a dynamic and ongoing event in the life of the staff member that should be shared and planned with the clinical nursing supervisor.

Clinical Conference. Clinical conferences are not a new concept, but often they are undervalued because of the time needed to focus a group discussion on a given client situation or a clinical condition for purposes of clinical management. One of the best ways to learn from one another is to share clinical situations and discuss appropriate interventions and care plans. It is always useful to have access to a clinician (either a nurse or physician) during these discussions as a way to expand knowledge and to consider additional clinical planning on behalf of the client. While one may think that the case presented at such a clinical conference must be unusual, the best learning happens in those situations that are common in any case load of the home care nurse.

Individual Conference. Years ago it was expected by both the staff member and the supervisor that weekly conferences would be scheduled and that these appointments were kept. It was during these discussions that coaching in the ways of clinical practice were formulated and plans for implementation were made. Until the staff nurse feels comfortable in these sessions, there may be some tension although this feeling should not last beyond the first month. The format of individual conferences is usually a tutorial in case management and case load planning as well as an opportunity to ask questions and explore methods of clinical practice pertinent to the responsibilities of the community and client home care needs. It is regrettable that individual conferencing has been dropped in many agencies and replaced with group teaching, or worse, no opportunity for coaching at all. The new staff nurse can encourage this practice in her agency if clinical conferences are not currently being held.

Case Load Planning. Educating staff members in case load management is a supervisory function that was once discussed primarily in individual conferences and now has shifted to group or team conferences. Managing client care requires identifying the needs of clients served by the home care agency and establishing an appropriate and timely plan of care. This is achieved most successfully in individual discussion between the supervisor and the staff member. It is not necessary to do this every day but, given that the average length of stay on the home care case load is a scant 2 to 4 weeks, it is essential to discuss and review care plans when the client is first admitted to the agency for care and every few days thereafter. Case load planning includes consideration of care by other home care providers, such as the medical social worker; physical, occupational, or speech therapist; and home health aide. Too often the staff nurse will discharge the client when nursing services are completed but other providers need to continue. Since the nurse is usually the coordinator of the client's care, it is essential in case planning to account for these providers and their work being done on behalf of the client.

Field Observation. Field observation is the tried and true method of assisting a staff nurse in the practice of home care nursing. When it is carried out well, it can be a most useful tool for teaching and for evaluating clinical performance. Often observation can affect the comfort and spontaneity of both the staff member and the family in their interaction. This can be avoided by having the staff nurse, in preparing for the visit, outline its purpose and expected outcome and discuss the extent to which the supervisor will participate in the visit.

A shared home visit is a variation of this supervisory method. In this case, the staff nurse and supervisor negotiate ahead of time about which parts of the visit will be performed by whom. Generally it is appropriate to plan field observations from time to time. Periodic field visiting with the staff nurse keeps the supervisor informed about the level of practice at which the staff nurse performs. As new technology is implemented in the home, it is useful for the supervisor to visit with the staff nurse and to learn about or teach the client about the new procedure. Conducting field visits with the staff nurse is the best way to initiate demonstration and return-demonstration of procedures or techniques of a skill and to observe the staff member's interaction with the client and the family. Most supervisors work weekends and holidays and must be able to describe a new technique or technology to staff members working with them. This is a good way for all parties involved to keep current on new and changed methods of care for the home care client.

Performance Evaluation. There are few activities that strike terror in the hearts of the staff more than when it is time for the performance evaluation. This need not be the feeling if the evaluation is developed as an instructive process during which plans are made jointly for facilitating the professional development of the staff member. Evaluation is perceived as a managerial activity more than an educational activity because it is often tied to merit or annual salary increments. A primary purpose of evaluation is to encourage each staff member to improve performance in the current job and to provide opportunities for workers to grow within the job. Too often, evaluation can be a litany of criticism and fault finding regarding past performance, or it is a glowing report of perfect performance. Neither approach is appropriate. The evaluation process should move beyond the past, which is a point from which to start but not at which to stop. Goal setting is the key to a future-oriented approach that stimulates improvement and growth. These goals should be developed by the staff member, and the supervisor should respond with ideas about ways to assist the worker in keeping the goals realistic and in achieving the stated goals. At the end of this section the agency's schedule and process for performance evaluation will be examined.

Problem Solving. Problem solving is often discussed as though it is a simple matter of coming up with the right answers. Actually, problem solving involves analyzing a problem and using factual information as a basis for examining it. The nurse must consider alternatives and implement the one that best suits the individual, the work unit, and the agency. Much supervisory time is spent in problem solving with staff workers, whether it is regarding assigning clients to staff workers, rearranging work activities, settling conflicts, thinking through a plan for clinical intervention for the home care patient, or planning and implementing changes in the work unit. The staff member acquires problem-solving skills for routine day-to-day activities in a fairly short period of time. The more complex situations, especially those of a clinical nature, take longer to grasp and will often continue to draw on the expertise of others.

Supervision of the Paraprofessional in the Home

The home health aide (HHA) is an increasingly significant worker in the home care agency. The new staff nurse responsible for the supervision of these paraprofessionals may not know how to work with, instruct, and supervise them.

A common pitfall for the staff nurse overseeing the home health aide is the temptation to neglect facilitating the aide's understanding of the care plan for the client and the family by limiting explanations to a series of tasks to be done. Like the nurse, the aide wishes to be challenged and given information to increase the knowledge base needed to care for the client. The supervisor can help the staff nurse to become better attuned to working with paraprofessionals. Although the home health aide may not have had as much formal education as the nurse, the nurse should regard the aide as a partner in the client's care, explain the care, and relate what needs to be done to the client's plan of care. The staff nurse must provide the aide with guidelines for observing changes in the assigned client's condition. Working along with the aide during a home visit can be a good way for the nurse to teach the aide and discover the client's personal care needs.

Some home health aides may possess only basic reading and writing skills. The supervising nurse must work with staff to develop communication methods that can inform the aide without causing embarrassment. This can be done through a one-to-one demonstration and return demonstration of a procedure or through pictures. Simple descriptive words are appropriate in this situation.

When English is the second language of the aide, it is proper to be sensitive to the manner and choice of vocabulary used to explain a procedure or activity in the home. Speaking quickly, especially on the telephone, is to be avoided and the use of body language when speaking in person is useful for more complete understanding. The nurse should bear in mind how she would feel if English were not her first language.

If there is any concern regarding the paraprofessional's literacy level, many cities offer literacy programs that can provide the home health agency with helpful tools and methods for dealing with this special situation. These tools can include some literacy screening material to help the agency in determining the paraprofessional applicant's proficiency in reading and writing and helpful guides to help the agency gear the wording on forms and records in such a way that the person with limited literacy skills can still communicate successfully. This points up the need for verbal exchange and for direct observation and review of the home health aide's work in the home setting to determine that it is safe and follows the nurse's care plan.

Supervised Activities for the Paraprofessional. It is the staff nurse's responsibility to supervise the work of the paraprofessional, usually a home health aide who performs some personal care for a client. Some home care agencies have home maintenance or home help services through which assistance is provided for doing some seasonal housework, such as washing curtains and windows and wiping cabinets. Other work done might include washing floors, cleaning the bathroom fixtures, dusting and vacuuming, caring for house plants, some shopping, and meal preparation. These activities are not supervised by the nurse The home health aide is supervised by the staff nurse after completing a required number of hours of training (commonly a 2-week, all-day intensive training program) that is followed by closely supervised field work. In 1990, Medicare regulations demanded that HHA competency and training measures be implemented in all agencies. Once the requirements have been fulfilled, the licensed and Medicare-certified home health agency can hire the certified home health aide. At that point, the aide is ready to be assigned to home care for periods varying in length from 1 to 4 hours. A longer assignment is possible but not typical.

The home health aide, one of the most valuable assistants to the home care nurse, provides much of the personal care for the client that is requested and then supervised afterwards by the nurse. The training that the home health aide receives and the continuing in-service education that is part of the employment arrangement reflects the direct supervision given by the nurse in the home.

The scope of work carried out by the home

health aide under the supervision of the staff nurse includes the following broad areas of activities:

PERSONAL CARE

- Bath—bed, sponge, tub, shower
- Hair care—shampoo
- Mouth care
- Shave
- Foot care
- Help with dressing
- Help with toileting—bathroom, bedpan, urinal, commode

ACTIVITIES OF DAILY LIVING

- Transfer client from bed to chair or wheelchair
- Assist client to walk with cane, walker, crutches
- Change bed, as needed
- Turn regularly, if bedridden
- Provide conversation, reading, crafts

TREATMENTS

- Take and record temperature and pulse
- Check and record weight and record
- Special skin care
- Measure and record intake and output
- Test urine and record results
- Remind client to take oral medications, drink fluids, eat
- Assist client with exercises as taught by home care nurse or physical therapist
- Assist client with elastic stockings, ace bandages
- Soak feet, special mouth care, special perineal care
- Feed client or assist in eating

HOME MANAGEMENT ACTIVITIES

- Marketing, meal planning, meal preparation
- Clean and tidy home (bedroom, bathroom, kitchen, livingroom
- Dust and vacuum living area
- Floor care
- Assist or do laundry, wash dishes
- Assist with errands, banking, mailing, and so forth
- Child supervision: bathing, meals, homework, recreation, bedtime

All of the above activities should be listed and identified on a worksheet for the home health aide by the staff nurse. The nurse can then acquaint the aide with the activities to be completed, and a worksheet can be left for the aide in the home. The staff nurse should evaluate the aide's performance every 2 weeks in the home to determine that the care is provided appropriately. Any changes in the care plan can be made at these times.

The care provided by the home health aide is essential to home care, and without it, the skilled nursing interventions necessary would be greatly limited. The clients receiving this care are often dependent on the HHA and are deeply grateful for this assistance, since they are often in a state of limited physical ability.

What Makes Supervision Fun

The part of the supervision that is exciting for the staff nurse and the supervisor is the noticeable growth that occurs professionally. This growth is expected. It happens in different ways and in different time frames, depending upon where the staff nurse is in her clinical development. It is rewarding to feel some evidence of clinical growth and leadership, when the staff nurse realizes her potential and reaches for the next rung on the ladder of professional advancement. It may not be possible for the home care agency to recognize the achievement made except to approve the recommendation of the supervisor at evaluation time for a merit increase in salary. There are other ways of recognizing good clinical judgment and practice among nurses and paraprofessionals. One is to develop an in-house ceremony for presenting a certificate or statement recognizing a particular situation where exemplary clinical nursing or home health aide practice made a difference. Another way is to nominate a staff nurse with an excellent practice record for a state nurses' association award or recognition for expertise in home care. Too often, the time is not taken to recognize, however informally, a nurse or paraprofessional colleague's work for a special intervention from which others can learn and for which all can applaud.

Clinical Exercises Common in Home Care

The Complex Clinical Condition

As a staff nurse of 8 months you are visiting a client who is homebound; in fact, confined to bed unless there are two people to assist her to the chair with the help of a lift. The son with whom she lives, is unable to manage the increasing personal care needs for his mother. For this reason, contact with her primary physician is irregular, and medical care usually takes place in the emergency room of the local hospital without this physician seeing her. Your clinical assessment determines that this client is physically compromised and headed for serious trouble. The primary physician agrees, in response to your call, that the client belongs in a long-term care facility. The physician states further that continuing home visits and requesting more help in the home (e.g., more aides, more equipment) only helps the son to postpone making the necessary plans. The physician then says, "I will not sign any more orders for home care services." You had not discussed this situation with your supervisor since she was new in the job (about 4 months), and you now need help. What do you do now? How? When?

Supervising Home Heath Aides

The district where you are assigned a home care case load has a large need for the services of home health aides. In fact, you realize that your home health aide supervision is increasingly hard to do in a timely way. You calculate that in a month's time, on the average, you must make about 20 supervisory visits. Scheduling them for when the aide is in the home, and doing them every 2 weeks is becoming a problem in planning. This, of course, is in addition to new admissions of clients, new home health aide orientations, and continuing visits for clients for clinical nursing care. You discuss your problem with your supervisor. What plans for supervising aides might you consider?

The "Special" Assignment Nurse

Your staff nurse case load is focused in the specialty areas of high-risk maternal–child health (MCH) care. You came to the home care agency with hospital experience in newborn intensive care, your area of expertise. This agency has not sought this client population in recent years, so it was necessary to build a reputation in the care of high risk MCH clients with providers who might refer clients to the agency. The intent was to improve discharge planning and to facilitate care in the home. After a year, this program was evaluated and showed minimal growth in numbers of referrals among infants and virtually no referrals of high-risk mothers. This is puzzling, and you wonder what you should do differently to secure appropriate home care referrals for this high-risk client. Meanwhile, because your case load is very small and you continue to attend meetings at different hospitals on the average of two per week, your daily productivity is minimal. You know your supervisor is concerned, and you decide to discuss this with her. What ideas do you offer?

Team Leader and Leadership

You have worked for this home health agency for 10 years, and you know your way around well. You have seen many staff nurses (and supervisors for that matter) come and go. Your supervisor rotates team leading on a weekly basis among the nurses on your team. The supervisor remarks that this is really not team leadership, but rather a necessary practical move for distributing the work for the day and to plan among the staff nurses which home care visits the licensed practical nurse might make that day. You are tired of this team leader business and resent having to take your turn. When you see your name on the list, you seem to forget to assume the task for the week, leaving everyone confused and angry with you. You decide to discuss the need to continue to take your turn inasmuch as you have seniority and should be able to be dropped from the list. Just as you think about this the supervisor calls you into her office for a conference and she begins with " . . . I'm troubled about the way you conduct yourself on the team. During the time you are assigned to lead the daily planning you don't show up. . . . ." Where do you begin?

Consulting a Clinician

As a staff nurse covering a district for home care clients you find that the cases are becoming increasingly more complex clinically. Several reasons explain this. Clients are discharged earlier from the acute care hospital; the people are older and more vulnerable as a result, and conditions that clients present with and now survive in seem to increase in number. You discuss your cases regularly with your supervisor, and one day she solicits your ideas about the need for some more clinical nursing consultation that might help staff nurses become better informed. You are not sure what this means and how it would be implemented. What you are certain of, though, is that this might be a reflection on how your nursing practice is viewed and you don't feel good about it. How do you proceed?

Time Management and Case Load Management

In any given week, your case load is expanded by at least six new cases. Of course, during this time, some discharges exist because of rehospitalization, recovery, or death. You find that much of your time during the first and often the second visit, is spent securing the necessary client signatures for various forms, reviewing the patient bill of rights, and checking the insurance, Medicaid, or the Medicare card for the spelling of the name and number that goes with it. Each signature requires explanation. You feel frustrated because you notice that so much of your visit time is spent on these necessary tasks that you worry that you might be skimping on getting a thorough enough clinical assessment upon which to base your plan of care. At your next supervisory conference you mention this to your supervisor and the two of you think about how this might be addressed and remedied. What are your ideas?

Productivity: Is it only numbers of visits?

You are seated in the office with your supervisor who lays out the previous month's productivity report. Your eyes fall to the bottom line and note that your monthly visit numbers and the year-to-date numbers seem to be inconsistent with the other staff. Too few. The discussion begins with that bottom line and immediately you feel yourself getting defensive and you decide to be careful what you say. As a result, you seek an explanation of the various columns (travel time, non-direct service time, preparation and post-visit time, etc.) to determine what all the numbers mean. What do you do next?

Finishing the Paper Work

Your desk is a mess. Papers are stacked, records have piled up, and a note from your supervisor on the top record says " . . . can't find the 485 for Mr. Jones . . . . the 488 is due today for Mrs Brown . . . . the visit made 3 days ago for Mrs Black is not charted . . . . " You go to your supervisor and say that you need help to get all the paper work done and submitted. You realize that no one can do this work for you and that with each day, you can easily get further behind, especially if you have to do paperwork for an admission patient. Now what?

The Motivated Staff Nurse

You just love your work and the variety of clinical situations you must attend to during your day with the home care agency. There is so much to learn and so many new procedures to do that your brain feels full. You decided earlier this year that you would subscribe to two nursing journals, and you pledged to read them as well. You are reading an article one evening at home about a procedure for drawing blood from a Porta cath, and you remember having heard a nurse colleague discuss this a few days earlier. You bring in the article and share it with the nurses (including the one who had been discussing it) and then post it for the entire unit to read. Your supervisor is pleased that you did this and comments about it to the group of nurses. A couple of days later your overhear a staff nurse say, "Yeah, you know she's trying to be smart and make us look bad because she gets those journals." You decide to discuss this with your supervisor at your next conference. How do you begin?

DEVELOPING SELF-SUPPORTING RESOURCES

Unlike other areas of nursing, the home care nurse spends much of her time independently, visiting clients in their homes. This means that there is little time or opportunity for discussion, informal socializing, or sharing clinical issues with peers. If a nurse is accustomed to hospital-based practice, this partial isolation may be one of the things that takes some adjustment. There are strategies that the home care nurse can employ to avoid the feelings of isolation and to foster professional development in home care nursing.

In many health care organizations, there are sufficient numbers of nurses working together to allow for informal socialization or collaboration. In home care nursing, the nurses may come into the agency for an hour in the morning and may or may not return to the office at the end of the day. Since the rest of the day is spent conducting independent home visits, there is little time for socialization or discussion of clinical issues with peers. The home care nurse should try to carve some time out of the schedule on a regular basis to meet colleagues for coffee or lunch. This is probably impossible on a daily basis, but once or twice a week is a good goal. If the agency has a regular coffee break time for staff before they leave for home visits, the nurse should try to attend. Interaction with all agency staff members can go a long way toward helping the nurse feel part of the whole home care agency.

It is also important for the home care nurse to continue to develop her knowledge and skills in the area of home care nursing. In hospital settings, many opportunities exist for impromptu discussions of clinical issues or informal in-service demonstrations of a new procedure. In home care nursing, these opportunities are not available and must be scheduled into the daily routine. The agency will likely have regularly scheduled in-service programs for nurses. The nurse should attend these programs even if they cover a topic with which she is very familiar, since this can provide her with the opportunity to refresh and update her knowledge and interact with peers. Home care nurses should try to take advantage of the many continuing education programs offered by home care agencies and colleges in the community.

In addition to in-service and continuing education programs, the nurse can remain abreast of current issues in the field through a review of the literature coming from the state nurses' association, the state home care association, and home care journals. The agency may have a central location where newsletters from various associations are posted. The nurse can ask her supervisor where those are kept and plan to spend a few minutes each week catching up on the current issues facing home care. If the agency does not subscribe to a home care journal such as **Home HealthCare Nurse**, it will be helpful to have an individual subscription to keep informed about the current issues in home care. These strategies are a few that will assure that the nurse feels part of the agency and cut down on stress. The following section gives another view of how the nurse can increase her knowledge about stress and how she can reduce the effects of stress.

STRESS IN HOME CARE NURSING

"If critical care nursing gets to the point where I just can't tolerate it and it's terribly unsafe, I may go into something else . . . perhaps community health . . . where there isn't as much stress or as many patient problems to manage. . . . " These comments were made by a critical care nurse who was interviewed for a television report in 1981, "CBS Reports: Nurse, Where Are You?" (Reemstma, 1981). While many things have changed in nursing during the 1980s, sentiments such as these are still very common among nurses outside of home care.

During the past several years many nurses have left nursing, complaining of increasing stress and burnout. Other nurses have tried to escape occupational stress by getting out of hospital nursing. For those nurses who have only worked in the hospital, many imagine home care nursing as a slower paced, easier job. Nurses interviewing for jobs outside of the hospital often assume that they won't have to deal with work-related stress, but most who take positions in home care find a whole new set of stressors. Home care nurses are burned out too, and many who resign from home care nursing describe occupational stress as a major factor.

The critical care nurse interviewed by CBS mentioned that there wouldn't be as many patient problems to manage in home care. True, patients in the community aren't as acutely ill as those in critical care, but she was probably unaware that most home care nurses manage care for a case load of more than 30 clients and, occasionally, as many as 40 or 50. She probably did not realize that home care clients in the community encompass all age groups and have vastly diverse problems. The assessment skills needed to manage these cases require knowledge of every physiological system, and in most instances the home care nurse does not have another nurse or physician immediately available to confirm an assessment or distinguish an abnormal finding. The specialty areas of the hospital are suddenly merged into one in the community: medicine, surgery, orthopedics, cardiology, pediatrics, gynecology, psychology, rehabilitation, geriatrics, oncology, and even opthamology (to name just a few!).

Home care nurses, expected to be highly skilled in assessing and providing care to a diverse group of patients, often develop additional skills as therapists, nutritionists, counselors, and social workers when these specialists are not available. The home care nurse is probably the only person who can change a dressing, prepare a sterile solution, order medical supplies and explain how they will be paid for, recommend a podiatrist who makes home visits, teach a specialized diet, arrange services for home meal delivery, grocery shopping, homemaking, and handicapped transportation, all during a routine half hour visit. It is no wonder that clients and families develop a real dependence on their home care nurse, since very few professionals in the community can provide as much skill, care, and information.

Most nurses who are new to home care bring some specialized skills, but they usually realize immediately that they have a lot to learn. Even nurses who have worked in home care for years usually feel they are still learning. Community resources are always changing, and the unique dynamics of each home care case continue to provide many challenges.

In order to feel prepared to handle the stress in home care nursing, it is helpful to know what specific issues in home care may be particularly stressful. How does the stress compare with stress in the hospital environment? Unfortunately, most nursing research on stress has focused on hospital nursing. Early studies on stress in nursing during the 1960s described the types of stress reported by hospital nurses, and in the early 1970s most of these studies were limited to intensive care nurses. In the later 1970s, research began to involve nurses outside of the intensive care unit, but even at the present time the focus of research on stress remains primarily on nurses working in hospital settings.

Studies on Stress in Home Care Nursing

In most of the literature "community health nursing" is the label used to describe what is also understood as home care nursing. Traditionally, the term public health nursing was also used, but in many areas public health nursing has recently developed a focus on epidemiology and disease prevention, as opposed to community health or home care, which focus on providing skilled nursing care to acutely and chronically ill patients in their homes.

One of the earliest published research efforts addressing stress among home care nurses is from 1983, when Jean Goeppinger interviewed a convenience sample of 36 community health nurses. Based on Goeppinger's research Tanya Case completed, in 1986, a descriptive study involving 61 community health nurses who provided narrative descriptions of stressful experiences. From 162 stressful incidents that were reported, Case identified 12 categories of stressful incidents in community health nursing. The categories of stressful incidents of community health nurses that emerged in Case's research were similar to those described by Goeppinger. The categories that Case described in descending frequency were

1. Political-bureaucratic problems ($n = 30$)
2. Understaffing and overwork ($n = 24$)
3. Interprofessional/interpersonal conflict ($n = 24$)
4. Difficult or unpleasant nurse–client encounter ($n = 19$)
5. Clients who are hostile, apathetic, dependent, or of low intelligence ($n = 15$)
6. Client's relatives who refuse or fail to deliver needed care ($n = 12$)
7. Unsatisfactory work environment ($n = 12$)
8. Inadequate communication ($n = 9$)
9. Clients who "fall through the cracks" in the system ($n = 6$)
10. Fear for personal safety ($n = 4$)
11. Difficulty locating client for care or followup ($n = 4$)
12. Miscellaneous ($n = 3$)

Comparing Stress Among Hospital and Home Care Nurses

Most nurses who are new to home care nursing have at least some hospital experience, so it may be helpful to compare the types of stress in hospital and home care nursing settings. At least two research studies have compared stress among hospital and home care staff nurses. In 1983, Nicole Hache-Faulkner, a public health nurse in Nova Scotia, Canada, compared stress among hospital nurses and public health nurses, using a standardized measure called the Speilberger State Trait Anxiety Inventory (STAI). The results of the STAI gave no evidence that either work environment was more stressful than the other.

Hache-Faulkner also gathered subjective information from participants using two open-ended questions. Think for a moment how you would answer these questions.

1. Please describe briefly a stressful situation that happened at work in the last 2 weeks.
2. Please describe briefly what two situations you find most stressful at work.

In responding to these questions, the nurses from the hospital and public health samples in the Hache-Faulkner study identified similar stressors, but they rated them in a different order. The order of most stressful situations for the public health nurses was (1) administration/management of the unit; (2) interpersonal relationships; (3) client care; and (4) physical environment. The order of most stressful situations for hospital nurses was (1) patient care; (2) interpersonal relationships; (3) administration/management of the unit; and (4) physical environment.

In 1989, a study comparing stress among home care and hospital staff nurses, utilizing the same subjective questions as the Hache-Faulkner study, was done (Cestari, 1989). Fifty-five (55) home care and 37 hospital participants provided descriptions of a recently stressful situation, and the two situations they found most stressful at work. The results in this study showed fewer similarities in the rank order of stressors among hospital and home care nurses. Hospital nurses in this study focused on staffing as the stressful situation most often described as a recent and frequent stressor. Home care nurses rarely mentioned staffing as being stressful. The issues that home care nurses seemed most concerned about as recent stressors were related to client aggression and noncompliance. Other stressors that home care nurses identified included relationships with physicians, work overload, political and bureaucratic problems, and issues related to the physical work environment and the safety of the nurse. Hospital nurses also rated relationships with physicians and work overload highly as recent stressors, but none of the hospital nurses identified either political and bureaucratic problems or issues related to the physical work environment and safety of the nurse.

Stressful situations described by home care nurses are interesting and often quite surprising. Nurses working in urban, suburban, and rural areas all described similar stressful situations related to patient noncompliance, which was the issue most often mentioned as a recent stressful situation. The stressful situations described by home care nurses included many comments such as, " I keep getting referrals on the same clients. No matter how many ways I try to establish a regime and help them become independent, they always drift back to their noncompliant behaviors. When they are readmitted, the ER wants to blame the home care agency for poor management of the client." Home care nurses also described stress related to aggressive behaviors by clients. "Several of my clients get verbally abusive when I try to explain that their demands for my agency to provide 24-hour care at home are unrealistic." Other nurses seemed frustrated by poorly coordinated efforts by other care providers. "If the aide doesn't show up the client calls me to complain, and I get tired of apologizing. Some clients have even gotten my home phone number. They seem to think I'm on duty 24 hours a day!"

Most of the concerns that home care nurses mention regarding physicians are frustrations when physicians did not call back, or were unconcerned or uninformed regarding client care management in the home. One nurse described a particular physician who refused to change treatment orders for wound care even though he hadn't seen the client in several weeks. Several others described physicians who made unrealistic promises to clients about the services that the home care agency could provide. "The doctor told the family that whatever he ordered Medicare would pay for." Situations like these often put the home care nurse in the position of trying to explain to families that the physician did not provide accurate information, something that families may not easily accept.

Stressful situations involving work overload are often described by home care nurses. When asked to describe the two most stressful work situations, the general issue of work overload is a frequent response. "Paperwork" is mentioned most often, with more in-depth descriptions usually referring to cumbersome documentation, Health Care Financing Administration (HCFA) forms, and poorly coordinated office support. Other nurses describe work overload in terms of their daily visit expectations and managing large case loads. As one nurse commented, "I have a heavy case load of very sick patients. I can't visit them as often as I should, because I'm so busy trying to coordinate care for too many patients, and there is no one to help."

Political and bureaucratic problems that are identified as stressful usually involve regulatory guidelines and paperwork. Nurses often described difficulties in trying to explain to clients why Medicare does not fund certain services or why services have to be discontinued at a certain point. Nurses are often uncomfortable discharging clients who still need care. These comments are echoed by many community health nurses. "Once the Medicare benefits run out we have to discharge most of our elderly clients. They still need the help, but there is no one to pay for it. I hate having to explain the system to people because I don't believe in it myself." The documentation required for Medicare and other insurance claims is also mentioned by many community health nurses as being very stressful. "I don't mind paperwork, but the documentation required by Medicare is ridiculous, and they keep adding more!"

Problems with communication in the work unit also concern home care nurses. These concerns focus on the inherent problems nurses in home care face by working primarily outside of the office. "It's hard to get to the staff meetings. I feel like I'm constantly back and forth to the office." Home care nurses often miss the peer support they have in the hospital with nurses on a particular unit. Staff in home care may come and go from the office at different times from day to day. Certainly there is more autonomy in this situation, but it is important to make time to communicate with coworkers.

Unacknowledged Stress of Home Care Nurses

When most hospital and home care nurses are asked whether they think their jobs are stressful, they are almost unanimous in their responses. Well over 90% say yes. Over 85% of hospital nurses also say that other nurses perceive hospital nursing to be stressful. Nurses in home care, however, often believe their work stress is unrecognized. Sixty percent of home care nurses indicated that nurses outside of their work setting do not feel their jobs are stressful (Cestari, 1989).

Why do home care nurses believe their stress is not acknowledged by their peers in other settings? One reason may be the limited exposure many nurses have to community health and home care in their nursing programs. Most diploma programs do not include a clinical rotation in community health, and many associate's degree programs cover community nursing only in theory. More and more bachelors of science in nursing (BSN) programs have had to limit their clinical rotation in community health nursing due to competing priorities. Student nurses who do have a clinical rotation in a home care agency may only spend 2 of their 6-week rotation in the field.

Student nurses who have the benefit of a clinical rotation in community health may not even develop an appreciation of the stressors in home care nursing. Nursing students often tend to focus on mastering technical nursing skills and may not have the time or inclination to become involved with the larger case management issues. The stressful impacts of work overload and enormous volumes of paperwork are often unseen by the nursing student.

Since little has been written about the stress of home care nursing, it is no wonder that many nurses tend to think that it does not exist. In an editorial in *Public Health Nursing* in 1988, Margaret Myers, a home care nurse, summed it up well. "The assumption is that the 'important' work is done in the hospital, and the visiting nurse might be sent in to just see that they're getting along OK."

Work Stress at Home

Most nurses who work in institutional settings, such as hospitals and nursing homes, are accustomed to being relieved by other staff members at the end of their work shift. Although the hours in home care often appear to be more regular, for many nurses the workday does not end when they leave the office.

A majority of nurses working in home care say that they *often* physically take work home with them, and most others admit to taking work home *sometimes*. Only a very small percentage, 5.5%, of home care nurses said they *never* take work home. In contrast, 32.4% of hospital nurses never take work home, and only 13.5% do so often (Cestari, 1989).

Because the volume of paperwork in home care nursing is intense and the case management issues can be overwhelming, most home care nurses seem to feel that they need to do some of their paperwork at home. Unfortunately, doing paperwork at home rarely allows the nurse to get truly caught up, but it may keep some nurses from becoming buried in a paperwork backlog. Inevitably, doing paperwork at home on a regular basis tends to become a habit that is not easily broken. The imposition of work into nonworking time often becomes a subtle stress, and the frustrations of work overload easily invade the personal time of many home care nurses.

Also, coworkers in home care are less able to pitch in and help each other than they would be in other work settings. Most home care nurses function in an ideal model of primary nursing. Many of their clients may not respond as well to being visited by different staff members, particularly the noncompliant clients who are so common in the community case load. It is also difficult for coworkers to help absorb paperwork from each other. Without being involved with an individual client, it is almost fraudulent to try to complete paperwork related to case management.

How to Handle Stress

The biggest overall issue that home care nurses identify as stressful is the broad issue of work overload. Certainly this issue is familiar to nurses in all settings, but the work overload in home care is somewhat different and is based primarily on the volume of clients that the nurse manages, the heavy volume of paperwork, and the subtle stress associated with managing difficult cases without the structure of the hospital or other institution.

Nurses in home care need to anticipate that they will be managing many more cases than they would have in the hospital, initially without much firsthand knowledge of individual clients. New staff nurses should not be expected to assume a large case load immediately. The most successful approach involves gradually assuming a case load, perhaps over the period of a month. Unfortunately, with recent trends

toward staff turnover, the luxury of time may not always be available. Uncovered cases may have been shuffled around among other staff members in the absence of a new primary nurse. All too often the new nurse is greeted with a large file of clients, with a barrage of phone calls and paperwork on clients she knows nothing about following. In any case, it is best not to expect to be familiar with all of the clients and understand their individual problems right away. The difficult and demanding clients are likely to make themselves known soon enough, and other staff members will surely be familiar with them. Do not be pressured into making decisions and taking action without the initial support of a supervisor or preceptor.

The volume of paperwork in home care takes every new nurse by surprise to some extent. The best advice regarding paperwork is to realize from the outset that it will never be all caught up. The new staff member who works late every evening and takes work home every night to catch up will likely find those solutions to be addictions; she will never be able to manage without taking work home on a regular basis. To some extent, the paperwork becomes more manageable once all of the forms are familiar, but it can still be overwhelming at times. Recently, many agencies have developed committees dedicated to revising paperwork and paper flow, and input from new staff members can be helpful. Committee work can provide an outlet and, in the long run, lead to some creative solutions.

Becoming an expert on all of the reimbursement issues and community resources, in addition to hands-on nursing skills, is an ongoing learning process. Most nurses new to home care find they are immediately more aware of current events and their impact on the community, especially legislative issues. Becoming active in the community is a natural inclination as the significance of social, political, and bureaucratic issues takes on a new dimension. For the nurse doing home care in her own community this role may be even more rewarding.

Many new nurses in home care look forward to increased autonomy and independence, and these are certainly welcome changes from working in an institutional setting. Very often, however, the autonomy can lead to a sense of isolation, especially for new staff members. If other nurses are being oriented at the same time, this may not be a problem. The new nurse can try to plan office time when most of the nurses seem to be in the office, either early in the morning or in the late afternoon. New staff nurses can learn much by observing how other nurses manage their case loads, paperwork, and phone calls. It may be helpful to find out whether people have a meeting spot for lunch, or whether there is another nurse seeing clients in an area convenient for meeting. Many home care nurses admit to eating many of their meals in their car, but it is a good idea not to get into that routine everyday.

Recognizing the stress in home care nursing is probably the biggest issue to confront in beginning to develop strategies to identify and deal with the stress better. In order to improve collaboration within the profession, nurses in all work settings need to develop a more contemporary view of home care nursing practice. This recognition can begin with nursing faculty in community health programs, who should be helping nursing students develop a more realistic perception of community health nursing—the good, the bad, and the difficult issues. Providing this foundation for all nurses, whatever their eventual work setting, will have many benefits. Exposure to the work stressors of home care nurses may begin to diminish the current sense that nurses in other settings are unaware that home care nursing can be stressful.

Nurses in work settings outside of home care would also benefit from additional in-service and exchange programs to put them in touch with the contemporary practice environment of home care nursing. Firsthand knowledge of the home situations, the chronic noncompliant clients and the voluminous paperwork and case management expectations of the home care nurse are largely unrecognized by other nurses. As discharge planners and hospital nurse understand these demands, there may be better discharge planning and referrals to home care agencies.

Nurses considering positions in home care should recognize that all nurses deal with stress in the workplace. Certainly there are many attractions to home care nursing, and highly skilled, sensitive, hardworking staff nurses are always needed. The types of stress faced by home care nurses are different, but so are the rewards. The combination of these challenges is what keeps many of the profession's best nurses where they are happiest, in home care nursing.

TEST YOURSELF

1. What are the three major expectations you have of your supervisor? What are the three major expectations you think your supervisor has of you?

2. Review your agency's schedule and process for performance evaluations. Discuss them with your supervisor.

3. What factors must be considered when supervising a home health aide?

4. What activities are home health aides allowed to perform?

5. What strategies do you think you will use to develop your professional role in the agency?

6. Ask a home care nurse who has been employed by your agency for more than 1 year what she identifies as the major stressors in her job. Discuss methods she uses to relieve those stressors.

Legal Aspects of Home Care Nursing Practice

OBJECTIVES

Upon completion of this chapter, the reader will be able to identify

1. Major client issues related to confidentiality and access to home care records
2. How home care nurses are accountable for their practice
3. Liability issues related to home care nursing practice
4. The process involved in a home care liability case
5. The various roles of the home care nurse in litigation
6. Several legal situations that can involve a home health agency

KEY CONCEPTS

- **Defensive strategies for home care nursing practice**

- **How to maintain a high level of professional accountability**

- **The various ways professionals are called upon to testify**

- **Legal implications of the home care nursing role**

- **What to do when served a summons or subpoena**

AGENCY-SPECIFIC MATERIAL NEEDED:

- Confidentiality policy
- Procedure for client to obtain home care record
- Policy regarding professional practice liability insurance
- Standards of care
- Policy or procedure for when employee served with legal papers

INTRODUCTION

This chapter has been included in the home care nurse's orientation to teach the ways that home care nursing practice will be affected by legal considerations. All nurses, wherever they practice, should be familiar with the legal ramifications of their acts in order to develop a way of practicing that is based on sound clinical judgment and consideration of the legal aspects of practice. Most nurses become anxious when approaching the legal aspects of practice, feeling that they would rather not know the possibilities of legal problems so that they will not have to worry. This book is based on the premise that the only way to prepare a professional home care nurse is to educate her to the many aspects of the field so she will be prepared to practice at a high level.

With this in mind, this chapter is presented in two parts. The first part describes briefly the many legal issues that are basic to the home care nurse's knowledge. The issues of confidentiality, the nurse's relationship to the agency, and risk management concerns, such as incident reports and insurance coverage are basic to nurses in all levels of practice. This section helps the nurse see how these issues specifically relate to home care. The material in this section should be covered in the first few weeks of orientation to the agency.

In the second section there is a more detailed discussion of home care legal issues, using as examples situations home care nurses have encountered. These situations focus around negligence, liability, and the role home care nurses may be asked to assume in testifying in a case. This section is included not to intimidate the nurse or make her fearful of home care practice. Rather, the thorough discussion of these situations, not so rare in home care nursing practice, can assist the nurse in understanding her role if these situations arise and help her to practice defensively in her everyday practice. This section should be used later in the orientation period and can serve as a reference for future situations. Appendix 4 contains a legal glossary which clarifies concepts used throughout this chapter and serves as a continuing reference guide for home care practice.

BASIC LEGAL CONSIDERATIONS IN HOME CARE NURSING PRACTICE

Confidentiality

The client has a right to privacy that is protected through various sources. One of these is the American Nurse's Association (ANA) Code for Nurses, which states: "The Nurse safeguards the client's right to privacy by judiciously protecting information of a confidential nature." (ANA, 1985). Exceptions to the rule against disclosure include the purpose of client care, disclosure for quality assurance purposes, and disclosure in a court of law when a client waives or lacks nurse–client privilege of communication.

Various state and federal laws also protect confidentiality of client information and records. For example, Medicare regulations prohibit disclosure without written consent of the client. The client may waive his or her privilege to maintaining confidential information by signing a consent form. Every home health agency should have written policies concerning the release of information in client's health care records, and the home care nurse should be thoroughly familiar with these procedures. Unauthorized disclosure could put the nurse at risk for liability to the client under the torts (legal wrong) of defamation of character or invasion of privacy. Defamation of character would involve publishing or disclosing untrue information that harmed the client's reputation. Invasion of privacy is an unwarranted exploitation of one's affairs and, usually, must be of a sufficient nature to cause shame, outrage, or humiliation for a client.

Every home care agency needs to have a policy on documenting the presence of acquired immune deficiency syndrome (AIDS) or human immunodeficiency virus (HIV) status in clients. Whether this is included in a part of the record that may be accessible to third parties, such as insurers, needs to be considered. Confidentiality of this information is the general rule, and release of this information without consent of the client (even to family members) could subject the nurse to legal actions by the client. Release of the information to others can have serious social, employment, housing, and financial consequences. The nurse should check her agency's policies regarding caring for AIDS–HIV positive patients.

Client's Access to Health Care Records

Although the agency has ownership rights in the client's health care record, the client has a legal right to the information contained in the record. In most states there are statutes concerning client access to health records that should be reviewed, since there may be exceptions to the general rule of access (Killion, 1985). The right of the client's ownership of the information in the record has been articulated clearly in court opinions as part of the common law. There should be a written agency policy regarding particulars of access for clients. For example, the agency does not usually have to provide immediate access, and the client may be charged a reasonable fee for duplication. The home care nurse should be mindful of the fact that the client may have an opportunity to read the documentation and recording should always be done in an objective and professional manner.

Clients should be asked to submit a written request, signed by them, as a prerequisite to releasing medical information to others, such as insurance companies that may have a legitimate interest in their health care. As an extra precaution, such written authorization should include the name and address of a witness to such authorizations, and it should be a part of the client's permanent record. In some instances, no permission is required to allow third parties access to the health care record. Examples would be for state licensing agencies, Medicare and Medicaid authorities, or to comply with reporting statutes, such as for communicable diseases or subpoenas issued as part of a legal proceeding.

If the client is incompetent, a guardian may be appointed in a legal proceeding to authorize release of the record. Even if the client is dead, the administrator of the client's estate can authorize release.

Access to the medical records of minors also presents a recurring problem. The agency should have a policy regarding this matter, but as a general rule if minors can consent to their own care under state law, then the parents will not have a right of access to the record. Examples could be if the minor was receiving services related to pregnancy, venereal disease, or substance abuse. Sometimes, if the minor is relying on parents for payment of the services, the parent may have a right to access. The administrator of the agency would need to check the circumstances in the particular situation and follow through.

If a client were to ask to see what the nurse was writing in the record, the nurse should talk to the client about the information rather than show the record immediately. Most often, the data will need to be interpreted in order to make it comprehensible. The nurse should use this opportunity to provide client education and information rather than hand over a copy of the chart to be read. Since requests to view the record are handled formally at the administrative level, the home care nurse would most often be informing her supervisor of the client's request. Usually when the client requests to see the record, it is a signal that communication should be strengthened with the client regarding his or her care.

Witnessing Documents

A home care nurse may be asked by clients to witness documents. First, the agency's guidelines regarding this situation should be consulted so that the nurse can follow them. A notation should always be made

in the client's record listing any documents that were signed by the client and nurse. Second, the nurse should record a brief statement on the client's orientation, state of mind, or any special circumstances. The nurse may be asked to represent the agency in having a client sign an agreement or contract for service. When this is the case, the nurse should ask a family member or another person to witness the document between the parties. This same procedure should be followed in other situations, such as when the client receives official information provided by the nurse when she is following guidelines set forth by regulatory agencies.

Occasionally, a home care nurse may be asked to witness non-service–related documents (i.e., those related to the client's personal business needs) that are not related to her role as a nurse. When a nurse does witness these documents, she does so as an individual. Therefore, a nurse should not then use the title "RN" with her name. A further suggestion is to limit participation by including the phrase "Witness to signature only" after the nurse's name (Connaway, 1985, p. 45).

It should be noted that the nurse, or anyone who witnesses a document, could be called upon to testify about the execution of the document. As a general rule, it is best to ask a family member or a friend to witness any service or non-service–related document.

Legal Implications of Employer/Employee Relationships

An employment contract setting out rights and responsibilities of both the employee-nurse and the employer-agency is a legally binding agreement between the parties. As such, this employment contract is enforceable in a court of law. To be valid, the contract need not be in writing and may be based on oral statements, but it is easier to prove once it is in writing and signed by the parties. Expected areas to be covered in the contract relate to working hours and conditions, salary, raises, length of the contract including notice of and grounds for termination, benefits such as sick leave and overtime, and vacation time. The position for which the nurse is employed, job expectations and duties, and types and frequency of evaluations should be covered. If any area is not covered in the contract that the nurse-employee feels should be included, it is wise to maintain some personal notes that reflect discussion on the issue.

If a problem should arise where either party feels the contract provisions are not being upheld, the first step would be to explain this to the other party. Written facts and specific instances should be used to support such an allegation. In the case of the employee, this may be in the form of a written performance evaluation based on criteria specified in the job description. Most nursing employment contracts are terminated by giving proper notice of termination usually within the length of a pay period or 2 weeks.

A second means of obtaining rights and responsibilities as related to a job can be through collective bargaining or unionization. This allows employees to negotiate collectively provisions such as salary and benefits. Typically, if there is a labor dispute, a formal grievance procedure is initiated, with specifics outlined in the collective bargaining agreement. Certain rights and responsibilities attach to these types of agreements as provided by state and federal labor laws.

Unless the nurse has either a contract or a collective bargaining agreement, the employer may have the right to "terminate at will." Recently there have been important exceptions carved out by the courts and state legislatures to limit this right of the employer to dismiss an employee without notice and without cause.

Employee's Rights and Duties Owed to Agency, Supervisors, and Board. Generally speaking, nurses have a duty to uphold the employer's expectations with regard to job performance. In home care nursing this usually means that the staff nurse should expect to be evaluated at regular intervals by supervisors. The nurse should expect these evaluations to be factual, objective, well documented, and substantiated by appropriate data. For example, if it is alleged by the supervisor that a nurse designs inadequate care plans, examples should be included. Employee evaluation data should not come as a surprise if the employee is kept informed at regular intervals. Employees have a right to evaluations that are made in good faith without intent to discredit or harm them.

Another duty the nurse has to the agency is to have standards consistent with the state nurse practice act and to maintain these standards through continued self-assessment and continuing education. The agency or employer needs to know if the staff nurse is unprepared to undertake an expected task. The agency has a duty to make reasonable assignments, consistent with the employee's education and skill. The agency, and ultimately the board of directors of the agency, has a right to expect notice from the employee of anything that is adversely affecting his ability to carry out his job. Examples would be if the nurse had concerns about personal safety or had knowledge of serious threats to the agency's reputation. Thus, even though there is no direct liability from the staff nurse to the board, the staff nurse provides information to the agency's administrative officers who channel the information to the board as necessary.

Another consideration of the nurse-employee is the right to view information contained in her personnel file. This usually includes any performance evaluations by peers or supervisors, letters of recommendation, forms from previous employers or educational institutions, or any disciplinary actions against the employee. Usually the nurse can review this personnel file in the presence of another agency employee, and she may have a right to copy the documents contained therein. Supervisors may have their own anecdotal notes to support statements in the file that the nurse would not necessarily have a right to review, unless official action was taken, and they became part of the nurse's record.

Evaluating Other Employees. The home care nurse may be asked to provide written evaluations of peers for quality assurance purposes or of employees under the nurse's supervision, such as home health aides. In the case of peer review, it should be clear whether the evaluation is solely for improvement of the individual's practice or whether it has implications for job status.

The same principles would apply as regards a supervisor's evaluation of a staff nurse's performance. In the case of the home health aide, the nurse is acting in a supervisory role and, thus, has the responsibility to judge the performance of the individual. Objective, up-to-date, well-documented, and ongoing data needs to be recorded to substantiate such evaluations. Included in the nurse's notes should be any corrective action (e.g., teaching a procedure again) that has been taken. As long as these evaluations or any subsequent letters of recommendation are done in good faith the nurse need not fear liability for these statements. Even if there are negative or potentially defamatory statements made (i.e., injurious to one's reputation), they are protected.

However, one is not allowed to make statements known to be untrue or to act in reckless disregard of their accuracy, or to act with malicious intent to harm someone by these statements.

Risk Management Participation

Risk management is a method of identifying, evaluating, and treating the agency's risk of financial loss. Most agencies are required by Medicare, accrediting agencies, or insurance liability carriers to maintain such programs. A well-managed program serves the interests of clients, employees, the agency, and the public.

Central to the operation of the program is a systematic reporting system of incidents or unusual occurrences with respect to any aspect of the operation of the agency. An example would be reports of frequent equipment failures that pose a potential risk. After a trend is established, an appropriate intervention could be carried out to solve the problem.

Staff nurses have an important function in reporting any incidents in order to assure that risks are documented and identified. The home health agency will have a procedure for reporting incidents and specific forms to be completed. Another level of participation by the nurse could be as part of an agency committee, sometimes a multidisciplinary committee, that reviews, monitors, and acts on risks. Individual participation in this process will continue to become an important area of concern by home care nurses in the future.

Incident or Occurrence Reports. Incident or occurrence reports are a means to report any unusual occurrence with regard to care of a client, and serve as a valuable record made at the time of the event, when memories are clear. An incident report is usually an internal document for the agency's use as a risk management tool, that is, through identification of areas of risk for clients, the agency can take preventive steps to avoid reoccurrence. For example, if there were several incident reports related to complications developing in intravenous administration devices for home care clients, in-service education for staff members and a better means of instructing clients could be instituted.

It is important that nurses recognize their valuable contribution in reporting incidents to help evaluate risks and potential liability for the agency. However, completing an incident report consistent with agency policy does not substitute for documenting the event in the client's record. For example, if a client falls while the nurse is ambulating him or her in the home, a brief factual account of what happened should be made in the record. Assessments and follow-up instructions or care should be included. There is no need to state "incident report filed"; doing so could lead a court to decide to incorporate the incident report by reference into the chart.

Generally, the incident report is not discoverable by the plaintiff should litigation arise over the incident, but this is changing, and some states do allow for discovery of these documents (Connaway, 1985). Incident reports should, therefore, be carefully worded so that they contain factual statements without admission of liability, fault, or how the incident could have been prevented. It is better to write the report in a manner that assumes it could be used for litigation. Some courts have taken the view that these reports are prepared for litigation and are, therefore, "privileged communication" or "attorney work product." Access to incident reports could help to substantiate a claim that the standard of care was not met. It is essential that all agencies have a clear policy for reporting unusual occurrences and that the nurse be aware of it.

Further suggestions by Nancy Connaway to help ensure privileged status for incident reports include having only one copy of the report, providing a checklist on the form to limit narrative comments, addressing the report to the agency's attorney or to the insurance claim manager, not using the incident report as a disciplinary tool, and not providing a copy for the client (Connaway, 1986, p. 10). All of these measures are designed to protect the confidentiality of these documents and to encourage the reporting of incidents as a risk management tool.

Insurance Issues

Individual Versus Agency Coverage. Considering the purchase of an individual professional liability policy is a personal decision for each nurse. The numbers of lawsuits against health professionals have increased dramatically over the last decade, with nurses being named as individual defendants in some cases. There are several reasons why it is advisable for the nurse to maintain such an individual policy.

Many nurses believe that their employer is responsible for any of their acts while the nurse is performing duties within the scope of her employment. While this is generally true, there can be exceptional circumstances. For example, institutions often have limitations in their policies. The new staff nurse can ask to see the agency policy and review it carefully, noting any exclusions or limitations to the policy coverage.

In some cases, a nurse named as a defendant may have to provide and pay for her own defense. In one such case, an RN anesthetist was named in a lawsuit along with her hospital (Sandroff, 1983). The hospital settled the case in exchange for a covenant or promise not to sue, a common right outlined in most insurance agreements. However, the nurse did not have her own insurance policy, and she had to pay for her own defense. Even though the jury returned a decision in her favor, she had to pay her own legal expenses.

If an agency pays a claim because of negligence of one of its nurse-employees, the agency has the right to sue the nurse for indemnification or reimbursement. Although not often used, the legal right does exist, and having one's own coverage would provide protection against such a claim.

Some nurses mistakenly believe that having one's own policy will increase the likelihood of being sued or will automatically trigger an indemnity suit by the employee, but there is no evidence to support this belief. In fact, it does not matter to the client bringing the suit whether the nurse has insurance The fact of insurance coverage or its amount is not disclosed at trial so as not to prejudice the jury.

Types of Coverage. Another limitation to the employer's policy could be the type of coverage. Many employers carry a claims-made type policy, which covers events that happen only when the policy is in effect. Thus, if the nurse has left the agency and a claim is made after her period of employment, the nurse will, most likely, not be covered. The home care nurse can protect herself from this situation by having an individual occurrence policy that provides for broader coverage. An occurrence policy covers incidents that occurred during any time period for which premiums were paid, even if the claim is made some time later. Another way to cover gaps in insurance policies is to purchase "tail" coverage. This could cover a gap created when a claims-made policy is cancelled.

Another factor to consider in deciding to purchase individual coverage is whether the nurse engages in nursing activities outside of her agency employment. For example, volunteer activities on a professional board, or as a camp nurse would not be covered by the agency's policy but are usually covered by individual policies.

Nurses are being exposed to greater risks of liability. As a professional, the home care nurse is performing a wider variety of highly skilled and specialized services. As an individual, the nurse can be personally liable for any judgment rendered against her. This means that if the nurse does not have personal liability protection, a judgment can be satisfied against her with her personal assets. Even if there are no current personal assets, future wages can be used to satisfy a judgment. With these risks at stake, it is unwise for a nurse to practice without individual coverage, especially considering the relatively low cost of such coverage.

It is still important to be knowledgeable about the agency-employer's policy even if the nurse decides not to purchase an individual professional liability policy. The amount of coverage, whether it is a claims-made or occurrence policy, and what exclusions or limitations of coverage are specified must be determined. For a thorough discussion of liability and insurance issues, see an informative pamphlet on **Liability and You—What Registered Nurses Need to Know** published by the ANA in 1987.

LIABILITY ISSUES IN HOME CARE NURSING

Negligence

Home care nurses, like all professional nurses, are liable for any harm to clients that is due to their negligence. Nurses are held legally accountable to a standard of care that is expected of reasonably competent nurses. The home care nursing standards of

care are discussed in chapter 2. The essential elements that must each be proved in a professional negligence or malpractice suit are

1. A duty to the client, or a standard of care
2. A breach of that duty, or a breach of the standard of care
3. Causation, including the fact that the breach of the duty proximately (directly) caused the injury
4. Harm or damage, usually in the form of actual physical damage to the client

If an injury to a client occurs that is alleged to be caused by a nurse's negligence, the client, as the plaintiff, may sue the nurse, who becomes the defendant. A major focus in the trial is to establish what the duty, or standard of care, was in relationship to the client's injury.

Sources of the Standard of Care

Nurse Practice Act. The basic starting point to define the standard of care for any nurse is the Nurse Practice Act, or state statute on nursing, in the jurisdiction where the nurse is a registered practitioner. Although practice acts vary from state to state, they usually contain broad language to permit a variety of activities by nurses. Many states have advanced practitioner statutes for nurses that apply if one assumes this role. It is important for the nurse to be familiar with the individual nurse practice act in her state.

Professional Organizations. Professional organizations or associations are another important source for the standard of care. For example, the American Nurses' Association (ANA) has established general standards of practice and a code for nurses, which outlines ethical duties. A Missouri case illustrates how the nurse's ethical duty is brought forth in a lawsuit (Cushing, 1982). The incident occurred in the operating room where it was alleged that the nurses should have stopped the surgeon before such extensive damage was done to the patient. In finding in favor of the injured party, the court accepted the evidence presented by the plaintiff that professional ethics mandated that nurses countermand a doctor's action if they feel it is incorrect. The duty of the nurses was to take whatever action was necessary to protect the patient.

Home care nurses must be particularly alert to the standards set forth in the ANA's *Standards of Community Health Nursing Practice* (1986) and *Standards for Home Care Nursing* (1986). For example, if a home care nurse fails to perform a thorough skin assessment (breach of duty) and the client subsequently develops a decubitus ulcer that does not respond to treatment (proximate causation and injury), the nurse's duty may be partially established through presenting evidence of standards II through V. These standards relate to the nurse's duty to collect data, diagnose, plan, and intervene, and they could be used to support a finding of liability for malpractice or professional negligence.

Other groups involved in setting and outlining standards for home care nurses include the American Public Health Association, public health nursing section (APHA); the Association of Graduate Faculty in Community and Public Health Nursing; and the National League for Nursing (NLN) (Northrop & Kelly, 1987). Regulations or guidelines established by these organizations could be relevant to the issue of what specific duty is owed to a client. It is imperative that nurses keep current as to standards set forth by these organizations.

Agency Manuals and Policies. Another source for the standard of care is agency manuals or policies. A home care nurse has a duty to follow agency policies and procedures that are consistent with accepted nursing practice. Two cases illustrate how failure to follow hospital policies has been used to find negligence on the part of hospital nurses. The same principles would apply by analogy to the home care situation. In the first case, **Czubinsky v. Doctor's Hospital** (1983), an operating room nurse left the first patient to begin assisting the surgeon for a second operation. This left only a scrub technician and anesthesiologist to manage the first patient, who was subsequently left paralyzed and comatose. The court held that these injuries resulted from failure of the circulating nurse and scrub nurse to monitor the patient properly and render essential aid. Part of the evidence presented by the plaintiff was the hospital procedure manual, which stated that the circulating nurse's duty was "to assist the anesthesiologist during the entire procedure." Thus, the policy set forth the standard of care.

In the second case, **Utter v. United Hospital Center** (1977), the plaintiff also prevailed on his claim of negligence against nurses who did not take any further action beyond informing the physician of the client's obvious untoward symptoms and documenting their observations in the clinical record. A policy in the nursing manual outlined a procedure for calling questionable care to the attention of the department chairman if the matter could not be resolved with the physician. The court found that the nurses had failed to comply with the policy in the manual and, therefore, were negligent, and the hospital was liable.

Implications for home care nurses are that the nurse should be aware of agency policies regarding how to deal with questionable care on the part of the physician or others in order to protect nurse and clients if a problem should arise. In all situations that the nurse may find in home care practice she must also be familiar with procedures and practices specific to her own agency. Since the site of practice is in the client's home, the agency has procedures for nurses to follow to receive guidance and support in questionable situations. It is the home care nurse's responsibility to be knowledgeable about them.

Publications and Current Literature. Texts and current literature in the field are other examples of sources to establish the standard of care for nurses. In **Guigino v. Harvard Community Health Plan et al** (1980), the plaintiff submitted a number of professional publications and newspaper clippings warning practitioners of the harmful effects of a Dalkon shield (an intrauterine device), relating to the time of the incident in 1975. The case was eventually settled out of court, but it alerts health care practitioners of the duty to review professional literature in one's field. A further illustration is the case of **Pisel v. Stamford Hospital** (1980), in which well-recognized textbooks and professional literature at the time of the alleged incident were used to help establish the standard of care for nurses. Expert witnesses, who were nurses qualified to testify on the accepted standard, stated how often the patient should have been assessed and what interventions were necessary to ensure the patient's safety. These experts used literature in the psychiatric field to formulate their opinions. In the absence of any written hospital policy, the court accepted the opinion of plaintiff's expert witnesses as the prevailing professional standard.

Expert Witness. In a malpractice case, the plaintiff must show the standard of care to be applied to the case. The usual method of introducing this evidence is to have an expert witness testify as to the prevailing standard. In fact, it is crucial that a witness who is familiar with the area of practice present an opinion. Both plaintiff and defendant will have expert witnesses render opinions when there is a question of professional negligence. In formulating an opinion, an expert relies on his or her experience, education, credentials, professional involvement, and any of the aforementioned sources for the standard of care. An appropriate expert witness to give testimony on a question of negligence in the home care setting would be a nurse who is experienced with the particular type of client situation, case load, and intervention that is brought into question in the lawsuit.

Testifying as a Nurse Expert Witness

A home care nurse may be asked to provide expert testimony as proof of the standard of care in a nursing malpractice case. In most jurisdictions, a nurse would testify on the proper standard of nursing care, although some jurisdictions would allow a physician to do so (Northrop & Kelly, 1987). Some states provide access to a panel of nurse experts through the state's nurses' organization.

The ability or competency of the expert witness to render an opinion is tested by the sufficiency of the expert's knowledge of the subject matter at hand. Expert testimony is admissible, and in fact necessary, when conclusions by the jury depend on facts or scientific information that is not common knowledge. Lawyers will seek the most qualified expert witnesses; Marie Josberger and Daryl Ries (1985) suggest that the following criteria be recognized in evaluating potential witnesses:

1. Graduate education in nursing
2. Clinical expertise
3. Research
4. Continuing education

The nurse-expert would review all written records, policies, environmental issues, and supportive management criteria (such as nurse–case load ratios), and pertinent literature to determine if the proper nursing process was followed. The nurse-expert would be asked to interpret these data and render an opinion as to the actions of the nurse in the particular incident as alleged in the lawsuit, usually involving a question of nursing negligence.

A home care nurse may be called as a nurse-expert to give testimony related to issues of child custody, termination of parental rights, child abuse, or criminal cases. Specific information regarding how to testify is provided in the section on providing a deposition that follows. The nurse can also refer to the documentation section in chapter 3 for guidelines involving recording these sensitive areas of practice.

Case Illustration—Negligence in Home Care Situation

The following case example illustrates several important areas of practice for home care nurses. In **Bass v. Barksdale et al** (1984), allegations of negligence were claimed by the plaintiff, an elderly woman whose treatment for tuberculosis was being monitored by nurses employed by the health department. The client was given a month's supply of medication to treat her tuberculosis by the defendant nurse, Barksdale. Thereafter, other nurses from the public health department made home visits and delivered monthly medications to the client over the next 5 months. The defendant nurse, Barksdale, who made the initial home visit testified that she dis-

cussed the client's medical history, informed her of the possible side effect of decreased visual acuity, and checked her vision with a 10-foot eye chart and recorded the readings. However, the client, Mrs. Bass, denied this. Interestingly, the eye chart Nurse Barksdale said she used did not have a 10/100 line, which is what she recorded for the right eye.

Mrs. Bass and her sister, who was present at the initial home visit, testified that Nurse Barksdale had forgotten to bring an eye chart and then checked her vision by asking her to point out certain objects in the room. Mrs. Bass also claimed she was informed only to watch for color changes in her eyes. The nurse who delivered the second month's supply of medication testified she checked Mrs. Bass' vision at that time. It was undisputed at trial that the health department nurses who delivered the medication over the next 3 months did not check the client's vision.

At a regular checkup with her private physician, who initially set up the treatment through the health department, Mrs. Bass testified she informed him of her abrupt vision decline. The physician denied she told him this. It was not until 8 weeks after this acute vision loss that Mrs. Bass went to an ophthalmologist who, through consultation with a neurologist, concluded that one of the medications she had been taking for treatment of the tuberculosis was the cause. There was uncontradicted expert testimony at the trial that if vision checks had been performed, her loss of vision could have been detected, the drug stopped, and her vision loss possibly could have been reversed.

In addition to questions of negligence arising in the nursing assessment and documentation for the client in her home, the case further illustrates the need for clear communication among all health professionals responsible for an individual client's care and for clear documentation of these responsibilities. Initially, Mrs. Bass' private physician telephoned the health department and talked with the defendant, Nurse Barksdale, who was charge nurse of the tuberculosis health clinic, about the care of Mrs. Bass. The content of the conversation was disputed at trial. The private physician believed that he had turned the care of his patient, Mrs. Bass, over to the health department, and at trial, denied prescribing her drugs.

Nurse Barksdale, on the other hand, testified that the private physician had ordered the drugs after she discussed the protocol with him. She further stated that then she asked the health department physician to sign the prescriptions, with the phrase "per telephone order of Dr. Schimerling" (Mrs. Bass' private physician) at the top. (**Bass v. Barksdale et al**, 1984, p. 481). The health department physician stated he never agreed to take care of Mrs. Bass and that signing a prescription form does not amount to assuming the responsibility of taking care of a client. The court agreed that even if the signing of the forms by another doctor was negligent, it did not create this relationship with the client.

The standard of care for a doctor prescribing the drug involved in this case, ethambutol, was established as including vision testing before prescribing the drug, giving warnings about the possible side effects, and what course of action to take if side effects occur. Based on the facts of this case, it is clear that a home care nurse should not ask a physician other than the one who prescribed the medication to sign a prescription form. Doing so can create confusion as to who is responsible for supervising the client while on the medication, and it can lead to serious consequences.

Another point revealed at trial in this case was that when Nurse Barksdale had Dr. Quinn, the health department physician, sign the prescriptions there were no markings on the "refill" line. However, plaintiff's counsel had been furnished copies of these prescriptions with "PRN" circled on each. Neither Dr. Quinn nor Nurse Barksdale could explain the apparent alteration on these forms. Routinely utilizing PRN refill for medications should be discouraged, since periodic rewriting by a physician would clarify accountability for supervision and monitoring of the client.

Another issue discussed in the case was whether Dr. Quinn, as the health department physician and therefore as Nurse Barksdale's supervisor, had a duty to ensure that she was acting competently with regard to the care of Mrs. Bass, that is, checking for side effects from the medications and checking her visual activity. Although the issue was not resolved in the case, the court stated that the jury could find negligence on the part of Nurse Barksdale and negligence on the part of Dr. Quinn for failure to supervise her acts. Although the court did not make a finding in this regard, the trial court's outcome was reversed, and a new trial was ordered to decide these and other issues.

Particularly in home care, there are areas of shared responsibility and accountability for physician's prescribing medications, and for nurses monitoring their administration in the home setting. Documentation of telephone conversations and their content, relaying prescriptions for physicians to sign after telephone orders are received, and documentation of client teaching and assessments will help prevent problems illustrated by this case.

Defending a Claim of Negligence

Pretrial Discovery. Before a trial on the issues related to liability goes forward, most states permit a period of pretrial discovery. This period of time allows for investigation of the plaintiff's claim and involves an information-gathering process. Through various processes, the plaintiff or client seeks to establish that he or she has a valid claim. On the other hand, the defendant, usually the agency or nurse against whom the complaint is made, wants to gather facts to demonstrate failure of the plaintiff's claim. This discovery process helps the parties evaluate the case and can facilitate settlement of meritorious claims.

The first step in the discovery process often is to request all records pertinent to the incident, such as the health care records of the client. Through review of these records, nurses who have knowledge of the incident are identified, usually through their documentation. A nurse is then identified as a potential witness for the trial. The right of discovery permits opposing parties to question witnesses before the trial.

Interrogatories. One way to seek statements from witnesses is to have them answer written questions called interrogatories. A nurse-witness should consult with the agency administrator and her private counsel or the agency's attorney about providing answers, since they are given under oath and need to be true as stated. Attorneys help their client complete interrogatories to ensure that objectionable questions are properly objected to and that the wording of answers does not suggest liability.

Providing a Deposition. A second means of obtaining information from a potential witness is through a deposition. A deposition is a witness' sworn statement, taken under oath that is admissible later in a court of law. The witness who is being deposed is questioned by the opposing side's attorney. Also present are a court reporter, who records all questions and answers verbatim, and the witness' attorney, who is there to object to irrelevant questions and to protect the rights of the witness. Occasionally, depositions are videotaped and can be used later at trial.

Being asked to give a deposition does not automatically mean that the nurse will be called as a witness at trial. It may be that the deposition reveals that a nurse has no significant knowledge of the matter, and this would end her involvement in the case. However, if a nurse is a named defendant, an expert witness, or a significant witness, the nurse's involvement will continue. The deposition is used to fix testimony for the trial, and it can be used to impeach the nurse's credibility, should there be differences between testimony at trial and that which was provided at a deposition.

At the time of deposition a nurse may be asked to discuss what she remembers about a particular incident. Copies of the medical record and other documents are provided for reference and review. Also, hypothetical questions may be asked. An example could be, "What should a home care nurse do if she observes that a cardiac patient is cyanotic?"

Guidelines for a Deponent or Witness. There are several guidelines that a nurse should follow when providing a deposition or appearing as a witness at trial. It is important to be prepared for the deposition or testimony. This usually involves meeting with the attorney representing the nurse to review the process, discuss anticipated questions, and review notations in the plaintiff's health care record. During the deposition information must be provided in a truthful and honest manner. A nurse should not guess at answers; just state simply "I don't know." Only information that is requested should be provided. The nurse as the defendant or as the deponent (one who is being deposed) is not expected to search for information that is not readily available. One should not volunteer information.

A nurse-witness or deponent is usually asked to comment or state opinions based on the clinical record. Since it is often years later that one is called as a witness, this underscores the importance of clear documentation at the time of care. The client's record, containing information recorded at the time of the incident, may be the only evidence of what was observed or what happened, since it would be difficult to recall solely on the basis of memory. This in turn reminds caregivers that documentation should contain facts related to what is observable and measurable. For example, "client looked better" or "wound improving" are nonspecific, evaluative statements only. It would be better to describe observable signs of improvement, such as skin color, vital signs, a measurable decrease in the size of the wound, or decreased measured amounts of drainage and what it looks like.

Sometimes the opposing attorney will try to intimidate a witness or deponent or try to put words in the witness' mouth. One should provide well-thought-out answers in a calm manner and avoid showing anger, defensiveness, or excitement. Questions should be repeated or clarified if they are not

understood. A deponent will have the opportunity to review the transcript of the deposition after it is completed and will be able to correct any errors or misstated answers. Throughout the deposition, the opposing attorney will be evaluating the nurse as a potential witness at trial, paying attention to the nurse's facial expressions, manner, and appearance.

Competency Hearing Testimony

All competent adults have the right to make decisions affecting their health care and other aspects of their life. This right includes whether or not they choose a recommended test or treatment and general control over their affairs such as to enter into contracts. Generally, state law defines a competent adult as one who has reached a certain chronological age, usually 18 or 21 years. Exceptions to this rule include when minors (under the age of competency) may consent to certain health care services, such as for drug abuse treatment and contraceptive services, or upon marriage when the minor is deemed competent to make his or her own decisions.

Thus, unless a person is found legally incompetent by a court, he or she is presumed to be competent to make his or her own decisions. The burden of proof to declare a person incompetent usually involves a showing of clear and convincing evidence, which is a higher burden than required by some other legal proceedings. When a person is declared incompetent there are serious consequences concerning personal autonomy and the right of privacy. Judges rely heavily on the opinions of nurses and other health care workers in rendering a decision regarding the person's competency status. If a person is declared incompetent, the court would appoint a guardian who would then make decisions for the individual. Nurses are frequently asked to testify at these hearings and would be asked to provide factual information, not opinions, as to the competency of the individual.

Another situation that the nurse could be asked to testify in with regard to the client's competency is a will contest. In this instance someone, usually a family member, is contesting the ability of the deceased to have made a proper and legally valid will. One of the issues that needs to be resolved at the will contest hearing is whether the deceased had the capacity to make the will at the time the document was executed. Thus, the individual's competency during the time in question is at issue.

The home care nurse may be asked to testify regarding her knowledge of the client at the time the will was made or changed. Relevant statements by the nurse include how the individual managed dressing and eating habits, household activities, and health care. If the client had problems in many of these areas, it could be determined that the client was unable to care for his or her person or property. By presenting this type of evidence, the one who is challenging the will hopes to prove that the deceased lacked the capacity to understand what the effect of the will would be at the time it was executed, and the will would be declared invalid.

In order to assess the deceased's state of mind, the testimony of nurses and others who had frequent contact with the client is invaluable. This can occur even if the nurse did not sign the actual will as a witness. Once again, documentation in the home care record assists the testimony. The nurse can usually refer to the record to refresh her memory, so detailed notes made on condition of the home, and the personal hygiene and decision-making capacity of the client are important. Any direct statements by the client concerning the will or business affairs should be included in the nursing notes since this could be helpful in any later proceeding.

If a nurse is asked to witness a will in the client's home, it is usually better to ask that someone else do this. Having witnesses sign a document helps ensure its validity and with some types of documents, such as wills, may be necessary to be legally enforceable. Taken at its face value, signing as a witness means that a nurse has seen another (the client), sign his name. This serves to substantiate that the person signing the document or will intended to be bound by what was signed. Witnesses serve a valuable function in any dispute that arises later regarding the will. The witness can give valuable testimony surrounding the circumstances of signing the will or document. Such proof may address issues related to forgery, duress or coercion in obtaining the signature, or the mental capacity of the one who executed the will (Connaway, 1985). Since a witness could be called at any time to testify or give information on these issues, it is considered prudent to have someone else sign as a witness. Some agencies have policies against home care nurses signing as a witness to a will executed by a client. However, this does not mean that a nurse may not be called upon to testify on the basis of her knowledge of the issues as based on the nurse-client relationship.

Guardianship hearings would be another example of a proceeding where a home care nurse could be called upon to testify on the issue of competency of a client. This usually arises when the ability of an elderly person to handle his or her own affairs comes into question. Again, testimony would center around the individual's physical and mental condition, care, and safety. It may be that the home care nurse notifies the family of the individual or a protective agency when there is sufficient information for concern. The court proceeding will then attempt to determine whether the person lacks sufficient understanding to communicate responsible decisions concerning his or her person, including provisions for health care, food, clothing, or shelter because of any mental disability, disease, senility, or chemical dependence (Northrop & Kelly, p. 270). Petitions to declare a person incompetent come from any number of sources, including friends, relatives, or health care workers. A finding of legal incompetence and subsequent guardianship can only be made by a court and should be distinguished from a physician's diagnosis that a client is incompetent. Sometimes, legally incompetent clients have been able to participate in decisions involving their health care.

In a recent New York state case, the right of involuntarily committed (incompetent) mentally ill patients to refuse antipsychotic medications was upheld (**Rivers v. Katz,** 1986). Wide latitude should be given to the client in participating in health care decisions. One cannot assume that mental or physical impairment makes an individual decisionally incapable. The right of the client to make informed choices is fundamental to the nursing care that he receives.

Activities Surrounding a Lawsuit

Initiation of a Suit. The first step in a lawsuit is for a party who believes that he or she may have a cause of action against another person to initiate the suit, usually through an attorney. The person who has the cause of action becomes the plaintiff and is sometimes referred to as the injured party. The defendant is the answering party and is the person against whom the action is sought.

In most cases there is more than one defendant named in the suit. A nursing negligence case would typically name the agency as a defendant as well as members of the nursing staff. Also included could be manufacturers of products or companies that supply products used by the nurse. There is usually a time period within which the suit can be brought in cases of personal injury. This time period, called the statute of limitations, is generally 2 years, with some exceptions, as in the case of minors. It is important that any malpractice insurance policy cover the statutory time limit period even if the nurse changes jobs or no longer practices as a nurse.

Summons. The next step is for the defendant to be served with a summons to appear before the court at a specified time. This process is known as *service* and functions to notify officially a named defendant that a lawsuit is pending. If a nurse receives a summons as a named defendant, she should notify her supervisor, her attorney or the agency's attorney, and, if appropriate, her liability insurance carrier. This is especially important since the defendant must answer the complaint within a certain time period or risk forfeiting the right to defend the suit.

If a nurse has an individual liability insurance policy, the insurance company may provide her with an attorney to defend the suit. This is a usual feature of most liability policies, and the nurse can review hers to check for this right. If not, the nurse should arrange to have an attorney of her own, since it could be that the agency's interest in the matter may be adverse to the nurses's.

Notice should also be given to the employing agency, usually through the supervisor, so that the agency's attorney can be prepared to represent any interest that the agency may have in the matter. Once the legal process has begun, the nurse-defendant should discuss the suit only with her's or the agency's attorneys or persons designated by them. Statements made to others may be introduced as evidence at trial and could be used against the nurse-defendant.

Subpoena. A subpoena is a document issued by a court requiring one to appear to give testimony on a particular matter. This may be in a competency hearing at probate court, child custody dispute, or a matter involving an allegation of negligence. A **subpoena duces tecum** is a subpoena that not only compels the witness to appear in court but also requires him or her to provide books, documents, or other tangible items in his or her possession that may tend to clarify the subject matter at trial. The nurse-witness should always check with her supervisor before supplying any such agency documents or client records. Usually when these requests are made, the person to whom the subpoena is served can request a fee for administrative costs or photocopying the materials. The person accepting the subpoena should promptly telephone the attorney requesting these records, so that payment can be arranged before any records are released. The same procedural step as to payment could apply when records are released to a client upon his valid written request, whether connected with a lawsuit or not.

It is important to remember that a subpoena must be complied with since it is a court order. Failure to do so may subject a person to being held in contempt of court. This is the reason for a subpoena; it is a formal process with a written statement delivered personally to an individual. In addition, the individual is required to sign that it was received, as proof of service. This helps ensure that the proper procedural steps are complied with as required by law.

TEST YOURSELF

1. Outline your agency's procedure for releasing information from a client's home care record.

2. You are on a visit to Mrs. Smith. In the home are her two sons and a notary public. They ask that you witness the signing of her power of attorney to the one son. What would you do?

3. What determines that an incident or occurrence report is filed in your agency? Fill out a report, making up a client situation, then review the content of your report with your supervisor and track where the report goes.

4. At work this morning, you were served a subpoena to testify in a competency hearing for Mr. Jones. What are the steps you would take?

Specialized Home Care Practice

OBJECTIVES

Upon completion of this chapter, the reader will be able to identify

1. The four areas to consider in the hospital versus homecare decision for high-technology care
2. The three main types of high-tech care provided in the home
3. Implementation strategies for implementing high-tech care in the home
4. The four reasons why there has been significant growth in the area of pediatric home care
5. The factors that must be considered before discharging a pediatric client needing high-tech support from the hospital to home
6. The home care services required to care for pediatric clients with specific illnesses in the home
7. The philosophical foundation of hospice care
8. The difference between traditional Medicare and the Medicare hospice benefit

KEY CONCEPTS

- **Nursing considerations for high-tech home care patients**

- **Ways of implementing enteral and intravenous therapy in the home**

- **Home ventilator care**

- **Preparing for the pediatric home care client**

- **Guidelines for high-tech pediatric clients**

- **The Medicare hospice benefit**

- **The philosophy of hospice**

AGENCY-SPECIFIC MATERIALS NEEDED:

- Policies and procedures for high-tech home care clients
- Client record and care plans specific to the high-tech client
- Hospice policy, procedures, and referral mechanism

INTRODUCTION

The rapid changes in the provision of home care outlined previously in this text have opened new areas of practice for the home care nurse. The provision of high-technology care, such as enteral and intravenous (IV) therapy and care to patients on ventilators, has created the new field called **high-tech home care**. This chapter discusses high-tech home care given to adult and pediatric populations. Also, the specialty area of hospice care for the terminally ill is discussed in the context of the home care nurse's practice.

HIGH-TECH HOME CARE

Historical Perspective

Home care has changed dramatically in the last decade, and several factors have played a role in creating the differences seen in home health care today. In the late 1970s, when the Social Security system was scrutinized closely, one thing was apparent—the current method of health care delivery, centered in acute care settings, such as hospitals, was costly, inefficient, and many times, ineffective. As legislators worked to find solutions, the manufacturing, health care, and insurance communities began preparing to position themselves favorably and safely in the face of new rules and regulations. Health care is a business, and like any other it had to change in response to these market demands.

So what were these changes in the market, and how has home care responded to them? The first change was the formulation and introduction of the Diagnostic Related Groups (DRG) system. In an effort to make hospitals care for patients more efficiently and effectively and thus reduce costs, diagnoses were assigned a number, a reimbursement amount, and a predetermined length of stay. The principle was that if patients were cared for well, they could be released on, or before, the predetermined time and the hospital would be reimbursed adequately. If the patient went home early the hospital made money; however, if the patient overstayed the DRG time limit, the hospital was financially responsible. Thus, efforts were made to have patients released sooner. No longer could someone recover at a leisurely pace as an inpatient. More emphasis was placed on families, friends, and health care agencies to manage the recovery period. The hospital became a truly "acute" setting.

Therapies that had in the past prolonged an inpatient stay such as IV antibiotics, pain control, hyperalimentation, and enteral feedings, now became a costly burden for the hospitals. Recognizing this, the pharmaceutical and health care products industries shifted their attention to providing these services in the home. Rapid advances in technology led to the development of lightweight, user-friendly electronic pumps for delivery of intravenous drugs by the lay person. Third generation antibiotics were developed that could be given every 12 or 24 hours, which made home antibiotic therapy more feasible. Insurance companies, recognizing that the daily cost of hospitalization, ranging from $200 to $500 a day, was eliminated with home care therapy began revamping their health policies to include home care.

The development of high-tech home care did not occur in a vacuum. A need was recognized, and many industries and home care agencies worked simultaneously to answer the need. As more and more clients experience these types of therapies in the home, there has been greater acceptance by the client community. The home care nurse has now become more specialized and needs greater training and expertise, especially in the area of high-tech care in the home.

This section will focus on what separates high-tech from less acute home care. Whether the nurse provides high-tech home care directly, works in cooperation with a high-tech provider, or refers a client to another agency, she will need to be familiar with the aspects of high-tech home care nursing presented in this section. In an effort to prepare the nurse at all levels of experience, a step-by-step approach will be taken.

The home care nurse is the axis of total client care, including high-tech procedures. The responsibilities can seem staggering, but by following well-established policies and procedures and using an organized approach, the challenge can be met safely and effectively.

The Hospital Versus Home Care Decision for High-Tech Services

The primary home care nurse is responsible for the initial assessment of the client, in addition to basic home care assessments. There are four areas to be evaluated when determining whether a client is suitable for high-tech home care services.

1. The client and family involvement with, commitment to, and understanding of the therapy
2. The safety and efficacy of the therapy itself
3. The availability of equipment, supplies, and expertise
4. The availability of financial resources

These evaluations are done before a physical assessment is completed, and any concerns must be addressed before high-tech home care is considered a serious option.

Client and Family Involvement. **The first evaluation,** although it may seem superfluous, is the client and family involvement with, commitment to, and understanding of the therapy. This is most important. Often, the idea to send a patient home with IV, enteral, or respiratory therapy is generated without much thought to all the people involved. The physician may face pressure from hospital administrators to discharge a patient who has overstayed his or her DRG time. The patient, himself, may be weary of hospital routine and wish to go home "at any cost." Or it may simply be that the discharge planning department views this home therapy as routine for this diagnosis and has set the discharge wheels in motion.

It is the primary home care nurse's responsibility to assess the client and family's understanding of the three **Rs** of therapy: the **Results,** the **Responsibilities,** and the expected **Risks** of their therapy. Ideally, a family conference with client, family, physician, and primary care nurse should be scheduled to discuss the three Rs. In reality, this is often not possible, and it becomes the home care nurse's responsibility to make this evaluation through individual discussions.

The client and family must have a realistic understanding of the expected **results** of the therapy, be it curative, palliative, or unknown. For example, a client must be able to distinguish between chemotherapy received in the past in hopes of a cure and the palliative chemotherapy that may be proposed at the present. It is equally important when the expected results are unknown or unclear, as in the case of pain control, human growth hormones, or some antibiotics, that any false hopes or expectations be brought to light and discussed. Using simple, direct questions the nurse can evaluate the client and family understanding of the expected results. Some of these questions are

1. Can you tell me what this therapy is supposed to do for you?
2. Have you had any medications or solutions similar to these in the past?
3. What was the result of that therapy?
4. What is your understanding of this new medication or therapy as compared with others like it that you have received in the past?
5. Are you comfortable /happy/ pleased with what your physician has proposed as a course of treatment?
6. Are there any terms, such as palliative, that you need explained in more detail?
7. What does the word palliative /curative mean to you?

The client and family must also have a clear understanding of the **responsibilities** involved with the provision of the therapy. All too often, physicians and other health care workers in the hospital leave the client with brief, surface assurances that the home care nurse will take care of everything, and "it will take only a few minutes (or hours) a day." Those involved need to realize that the time commitment to high-tech home care can often be restrictive. They must also recognize and be prepared for the client's shift in dependence from hospital personnel to family, friends, and home health agency personnel.

The most effective way to help clients realize these responsibilities is to outline for the client and family what a typical 24-hour period will be like with their therapy. It is important to tie aspects of the therapy into their individual daily lives and routines. For example, "Mrs. Jones, you will be giving your mother the antibiotic at 8:00 AM and 8:00 PM daily. You will need to begin preparing your supplies at 7:45 so that you can start on time. The infusion takes 30 minutes so that at 8:15 you will have to assemble all your disconnection supplies. You will need to plan to be involved with this whole process from 7:45 AM to 8:45 AM. Knowing this will allow you to plan enough time to get ready for work. The therapy is scheduled for a month and one-half (6 weeks)." By giving those involved time frames as they relate to their own daily routines and schedules, there is less chance for feelings of disillusionment and frustration with the therapy.

The final R is the **risks** of therapy, and this is both an important and delicate subject. The risks of each type of therapy should first be discussed with the physician and home health manager responsible for this function. A word of caution, all clients are entitled to be informed of all risks involved in their therapy. It is also important to indicate the risks inherent in the delivery of therapy at home versus the hospital. In reality, however, a physician or family member may wish that certain risks be deemphasized. This is not a decision that the primary nurse should make. It is, however, one that should be discussed with the physician and nursing supervisor and, as indicated, other family members.

The home care nurse's responsibility in assessing the client and family understanding of the three Rs is imperative to successful therapy. The nurse must feel confident that they clearly understand what the therapy is for, how much they will be doing, and what risks they accept as part of the therapy.

Safety and Efficacy of the Therapy. **The second evaluation** area is the safety and efficacy of the therapy itself. This is independent of the client's understanding of risk factors. Safety factors include the environment in which the therapy will be provided, both physical and emotional, side effects and effects of the medications or solutions, and the functional ability of the client or caregiver who will be performing the procedures.

For example, in pain control therapy there must be a caregiver who is physically and emotionally able to deliver the medication. The client, under the influence of a narcotic, is neither physically or mentally able to safely perform the necessary procedures. A close family relative, such as a spouse, may be emotionally incapable of safely adjusting narcotic doses or accepting the client's response to narcotic therapy.

Another safety factor involves the expected effects or side effects of the medications or equipment. For example, the side effects of amphotericin B include hypotension, fever spikes, and cardiac arrhythmias which are often unpredictable and may require emergency intervention. A successful course of treatment in the hospital does not ensure the same at home. This may be an innapropriate therapy based on the safety risks inherent in the therapy itself. With regard to equipment, a home respirator in a house with old or unsafe wiring may also be innapropriate.

And finally, a more subtle and often overlooked safety factor is the ease with which a therapy can be delivered in the home. The goal in home care is to teach the client and family to be independent in the client's care. Since mechanical and electronic equipment are often required, it is imperative that the client and family are able to learn how to use and troubleshoot the equipment. For example, hyperalimentation therapy with concomitant pain control and chemotherapy require the use of several pumps and numerous solution changes daily. When the demands of the therapy are so complex as to convert the home to a hospital it may be that the hospital is, in reality, a safer and more economical choice. The complexity of this therapy regime may be far beyond the ability of most family members. To summarize, the safety and efficacy of the therapy must be evaluated based on the equipment being used, the mental, emotional, and physical abilities of those involved, and risk factors of the therapy, medication, or equipment.

Availability of Equipment and Expertise. The third major evaluation area is the availability of equipment and expertise. When the therapy is initially mapped out, the primary nurse will need to determine whether it is possible to deliver the therapy as ordered. Specifically, in reviewing the therapy orders the nurse must determine what equipment and how much support personnel at what skill level will be necessary. There are still limitations to current technology. For example, the small portable pumps can deliver fluid only in amounts ranging from 10 cc to 250 cc. Therefore, a 2-g dose of vancomycin to be given in 500 ml of solution would not be appropriate for a portable pump. The question then becomes, is a large stationary pump acceptable and feasible for the client's life-style? Modifications may be necessary if the client was planning to administer therapy while in the workplace.

The availability of expertise is as important as the availability of equipment. There must be a caregiver or outside support personnel able to perform the necessary procedures or provide backup. With relation to personnel, the nurse must assess (1) Does this case require additional professional help, such as oncology or pediatrics; (2) Are these specialists available at the times of the day and night when the client needs them? (3) Does the family need full or partial support? (4) Are the outside personnel available in the client's geographic area? All of these questions must be answered before a determination can be made about the feasibility of providing the therapy in the home. It is, again, the primary nurse's responsibility to assess whether this therapy can be safely and effectively provided with the equipment and personnel available.

Financial Resources. The fourth and final area to be evaluated, financial coverage, is an equally important factor. Many nurses find dealing with insurance companies, clients, and government agencies regarding finances difficult. The home care nurse, however, can be the critical factor that determines whether a therapy will be covered. Consider what goes into the coverage decision. It is important to understand that insurance companies have rigid coverage guidelines and that the representatives encountered will be clerical employees. At this stage it is best to ask broad questions and listen well.

The nurse should identify herself and indicate that she is calling for the client. She should explain that she has some questions regarding the client's insurance coverage for home care. Have all pertinent information readily available. The following information is essential:

1. Client's name
2. Subscriber's name (in whose name the insurance is carried)
3. Policy number
4. Social security number of client and subscriber
5. Subscriber's employer
6. Client diagnosis
7. Type of therapy
8. Expected duration of therapy
9. Equipment needed
10. Support personnel needed

Initial questions should be similar to the following:

1. Does Mrs. Smith have home care coverage in her policy?
2. Does this policy include intravenous (enteral, respiratory) therapy?
3. Are RNs, LPNs, and other therapists covered under this policy?
4. What, if any, are the restrictions to this coverage?

All answers should be carefully documented. Answers will come in various forms, such as "intravenous therapy is covered only when it is deemed medically necessary." Ask for their definition of medically necessary and inquire as to what proof they require (e.g., physician's letter, a hospital document, a determination by *their* medical review board).

When determining coverage for nursing service, the answer may be "the patient is allowed 40 visits per calendar year." It is important to ask how the insurance provider defines a visit (an hour, or a 4- to 8-hour block of time). Can there be more than one visit per day? Does the insurer pay for visits exceeding the 40? Has the client used any visits within the current calendar year?

After the nurse has the answers to these questions she can ask for an RN case manager or reviewer. Many insurance companies have created these positions to review the "appropriateness" of care. At this point, talking with a professional peer, the home care nurse can discuss and clarify the coverage issues without being afraid or intimidated. The client has a right to utilize the benefits paid for to the fullest, and home care can be a cost-effective alternative.

The discussion should begin with a review of the client's coverage and be followed by the nurse's conclusion, such as "Based on Mrs. Smith's coverage it is safe to assume that her 4-week course of antibiotic therapy is covered. She will require daily visits by an RN, equaling 28 days this calendar year, out of her allowed 40. In addition, it is my understanding that only a portable, electronic pump is covered and that all drugs and biologicals will be covered at 100%." The discussion is concluded by clarifying what paperwork the insurance company requires, usually physician's orders, nurse's notes, a letter of medical necessity, and any forms specific to the insurance company.

The date and time of the conversation and the full names of all personnel spoken with should be documented carefully in the client's record, and it is useful to have these benefits confirmed in writing. With the coverage information in hand, the nurse can discuss with the client, family, and physician whether to proceed with the therapy.

The decision to provide therapy in the home in lieu of hospitalization is often not a simple one. Completing a step-by-step assessment of the feasibility of home care *before* the client goes home will assure a more successful course of therapy. To review, the four major areas to consider are

1. Client and family involvement
2. Safety and efficacy of therapy
3. Availability of equipment and expertise
4. Financial resources

All of these must work together to assure success of the client's home care and be reviewed *before* the client is discharged.

Types of High-Tech Home Care

Presently, there is no concrete definition of what constitutes high-tech home care. For the purposes of this section, the focus will be on three areas: enteral therapy, intravenous therapy, and home ventilation. Table 7–1 lists common diagnoses requiring one or more of these therapies in the home.

Enteral Therapy. Enteral therapy involves the provision of nutrients through a tube resting in the gut. This can be a nasogastric, gastric, or jejunostomy tube. Feedings consist of highly concentrated solutions containing the carbohydrates, proteins, vitamins, minerals, and electrolytes necessary to sustain life. Enteral therapy is most commonly used for clients with obstructions or malabsorption syndromes or clients with increased nutritional needs. The placement of the tube is dependent on the length of therapy and the condition of the intestinal tract.

Enteral therapy is provided either by bolus method, continuous drip, or a modified combination of the two. Nursing considerations relate to

1. The placement and integrity of the tube
2. The client's tolerance of the solution
3. The client's acceptance of the diagnosis and enteral therapy routine
4. The client's fluid and electrolyte balance

This therapy is perhaps the easiest to provide in the home since the procedure itself is simple and easily taught to both client and family. In addition, it is readily covered by insurance carriers, including Medicare. It is important to remember that to assure coverage, the primary diagnosis must *justify* the need for enteral feedings. For example, although the client's primary diagnosis may be cancer, the home care diagnosis must describe the condition creating the need for enteral feedings, such as bowel obstruction or malabsorption syndrome.

Although teaching the client and family is the nurse's primary focus of care for the client with enteral therapy, the responsibility of the primary care

TABLE 7–1. DIAGNOSES FOR HOME THERAPIES

HOME ANTIBIOTIC THERAPY		
Abscesses	Cystic fibrosis	Prostatitis
AIDS-Related Opportunistic Infections	Fungal infections (local and systemic)	Pyelonephritis
Acute leukemia	Infected orthopedic appliances	Sepsis
Bacteremia	Otitis media	Septic arthritis
Bacterial endocarditis	Osteomyelitis	Sinusitis
Candidal endocarditis	Pelvic inflammatory disease	Wound infections
Cellulitis	Peritonitis	
Chronic urinary tract infections	Pneumonia	

HOME PARENTERAL NUTRITION		
AIDS-related enteropathy	Congenital bowel malformation	Malabsorption
Biliary atresia	Crohn's disease	Malnutrition
Biliary cirrhosis	Cystic fibrosis	Mesenteric infarction
Bowel obstruction	Enterocutaneous fistula	Metabolic disorders
Cancer of the abdomen	Failure to thrive	Pancreatitis
Cancer of the bladder	Gastroenteritis	Post-op–Pre-op nutritional support
Cancer of the colon	Hirschsprung's disease	Pseudo-obstruction
Cancer of the liver	Hyperemesis gravidarum	Radiation enteritis
Cancer of the pancreas	Inflammatory bowel disease	Scleroderma of the GI tract
Cancer of the stomach	Intractable diarrhea	Short bowel syndrome
Chronic renal failure	Ischemic bowel disease	Sprue
Colitis		

HOME ENTERAL NUTRITION		
Achalasia	Cerebral vascular accident	Inflammatory bowel disease
Anorexia	CNS diseases that impair swallowing	Intestinal atresia
Biliary atresia	Colitis	Intractable diarrhea
Biliary cirrhosis	Congenital abnormalities of GI tract	Ischemic bowel disease
Cachexia	Cystic fibrosis	Malnutrition
Cancer of the head or neck	Dysphagia	Motility disorders
Cancer of the pharynx	Esophageal stricture	Pancreatitis
Cancer of the esophagus	Failure to thrive	Pseudo-obstruction
Cancer of the stomach	Fistula	Short bowel syndrome
Cancer of the pancreas	Gastroenteritis	Sprue

HOME CONTINUOUS CHEMOTHERAPY		

Carcinomas of
    breast, esophagus, lung, pancreas, GI
    tract (colorectal, anal, gastric), head
    and neck, lung, cervix, ovaries,
    testicles
	Germ cell neoplasms
	Histoplasmosis
	Leukemias
	Lymphomas
	Sarcomas
		Small cell carcinoma of the lung
		Squamous cell carcinoma of the cervix,
		    head, or neck

HOME PAIN MANAGEMENT		
Chronic intractable pain secondary to Carcinomas and lymphomas	AIDS-related diagnoses	End-stage cardiac disease

HOME HYDRATION THERAPY		

Fluid & eletrolyte imbalance secondary to
    Gastrointestinal dysfunction
    Gastroenteritis
	Hyperemesis gravidarum
	Intractable diarrhea
		Short bowel syndrome

From: Med-Center Home Health Care Inc; Danbury CT, with permission.

nurse does not end with teaching. Table 7–2 summarizes the common complications of enteral therapy. The home care nurse's teaching tools should clearly show the client and family how to assess for possible complications, and documentation must reflect both this teaching and the nurse's own skilled observation of the client as they relate to these possible complications. Periodic reassessments should be made, as a client may initially tolerate enteral therapy and not display signs of complication until several weeks or months have passed.

Intravenous Therapy. Intravenous (IV) therapy is the broadest category in high-tech home care. The five

TABLE 7–2. GASTROINTESTINAL COMPLICATIONS OF ENTERAL NUTRITION SUPPORT

Signs & Symptoms	Possible Causes	Management
Diarrhea	—Dumping Syndrome	1. Dilute nutrient 2. Reduce rate of administration 3. Consider continuous infusion rather than bolus 4. Consider use of antidiarrheal drugs
Nausea Vomiting	—Nutrient source too concentrated —Rate of administration too rapid	1. Dilute nutrient 2. Reduce rate of administration 3. Consider continuous infusion rather than bolus 4. Consider alternate enteral formula (lactose free, medium chain triglycerides) 5. Consider supplemental use of intravenous support
Bloating Cramping	—Rate of administration of nutrient mixture is too rapid —Fat intolerance	1. Reduce rate of administration 2. Consider continuous infusion rather than bolus
Hypermotility Distention	—Malabsorption —Fat intolerance —Nutrient source too concentrated —Rate of administration too rapid	1. Reduce rate of administration 2. Consider alternate enteral formula 3. Dilute nutrient concentration
Flatulence Borborygmus	—Fat intolerance —Lactose deficiency	1. Consider alternate enteral formula 2. Reduce concentration

From: Med-Center Home Health Care Inc; Danbury, CT, with permission.

major types of IV therapy are antibiotic, pain control, hyperalimentation, hydration, and chemotherapy Less common therapies include human growth hormones, cardiac drugs, blood and blood components and aminophylline therapy.

Intravenous therapy is provided either peripherally or via a central line access. The myriad types of peripheral access cannot be reviewed individually in this text. The common heplock is currently the most widely used access. For longer peripheral placement, the Pik Line is currently being utilized. The home care nurse should familiarize herself with the devices used in the area hospitals from which she receives client referrals.

Central access lines are of two main types: Hickman/Broviac and Port-a-Cath. Like peripheral lines, the variety of central lines is too great to list. The Hickman/Broviac is a cuffed central line that is placed in the chest or abdominal wall by blunt dissection. The tip is threaded through a major vessel, usually the brachial artery, into the superior vena cava where it rests just outside the atrium. The Port-a-Cath is placed in the same manner. The external end of the Hickman/Broviac protrudes approximately 6 to 12 inches from the exit wound. Within the first 3 to 10 postoperative days, wound healing occurs around the catheter cuff creating a "natural" barrier to infection. The Port-a-Cath does not have an external apparatus. Instead, the "port" is placed under a skin flap in the chest wall, much like a pacemaker. The line is accessed utilizing a special curved, non-

boring Huber needle, which pierces the skin and face of the port. The needle is held in place by an occlusive dressing. The port is normally reaccessed once weekly, or more frequently depending on the therapy.

Hydration and antibiotic therapies are commonly given via a peripheral line. Chemotherapy, pain control, and hyperalimentation are almost exclusively given through a central access. Appendix 5 lists the drugs and solutions most commonly used in home care.

Rapid advances in technical research and design have produced a large variety of small, lightweight pumps for use in all types of intravenous therapy Examples of syringe style pumps include the Auto Syringe and Becton Dickinson. Examples of pumps that utilize a cassette type reservoir are the Cadd 5100 and the Cadd PCA 5200 pumps. A third style of portable pumps allows for the use of 50, 100, and 250 cc minibags, such as the Pancreatic pump and the Parker infuser. Recently developed nonmechanical pumps, such as the Travenol Infuser and the Intermate, are lightweight, disposable, and easy to use.

The primary care nurse must choose the most appropriate pump for the client and therapy. The pharmacist and pharmaceutical company nurse are often excellent resources to assist in making this decision. As a general rule, pain control and chemotherapy should always be given in a cassette style pump with computerized locking mechanisms for the dose and rate. This assures accurate dosage while preventing accidental or intentional tampering. Syringe and minibag style pumps and nonmechanical infusers are all appropriate for use in peripheral antibiotic therapy.

In order to choose the correct pump, the following information must be assessed:

1. What is the volume of solution or medication to be delivered?
2. Over what time period? (Hours, days)
3. For how long, once reconstituted, is the medication stable? (Hours, days, weeks)
4. Does the therapy require a constant rate and dosage or does the rate or dose vary?
5. What is the learning and functional ability of the client or caregiver who is going to be taught the use of the pump?

With this information, a comparison can be made of the pumps available. The correct pump should be appropriate for the learner, have the capacity for the volume of solution, and have features that provide the safe and efficient administration of the required medication.

Hyperalimentation should be provided exclusively via a stationary pump, such as a HomePro, Travenol 6100, or Imed. Like the portable pumps, each of these was designed with specific features for safe, effective delivery of solutions. For example, the HomePro pump has a programmable tapering feature to establish an easing on and tapering off schedule for TPN that is given on a rotating schedule (e.g., 12 hours on, 12 hours off).

The HomePro automatically increases slowly the rate at the beginning and decreases it at the end of the infusion time. This reduces the incidence of rapid blood sugar fluctuation in the client.

In order to provide IV and enteral therapy in the home the nurse must locate and familiarize herself with resources for the following:

1. Compatibility and stability information for enteral and parenteral solutions commonly used in home care
2. Acceptable diagnosis for each type of therapy
3. Pump specification and features for pumps used by the home health agency
4. Policies and procedures for administration of each type of therapy

Home Ventilator Care. The final category of high-tech care is home ventilator care. Unlike the other types of home therapy for which the nurse will act as the primary coordinator, in home ventilator therapy the respiratory therapist will function in this capacity. Most respiratory therapy companies have very strict policies and procedures under which they function. It is helpful for the nurse to obtain a copy of these and

be familiar with them. The information outlined in the following paragraphs is based on general guidelines common to many companies.

The initial assessment of the client to determine whether he or she is a candidate for home ventilator therapy will include physiological, sociological, mental, and emotional evaluations. The client must have 24-hour attendance at all times either by the family or qualified support personnel, and there must be a physician and registered respiratory therapist available on-call at all times. The home must meet all the electrical and structural requirements of the company providing the respiratory equipment, as well as back-up measures, such as a generator in case of power failure.

Training for ventilator therapy always occurs in the hospital setting. The hospital usually accepts responsibility for training the primary care provider the elements of client care, including suctioning, tracheostomy tube cleaning and changing, cardiopulmonary resuscitation (CPR), and general client body care. The care and functioning of the ventilator itself is most often taught by the company's respiratory therapist. If the model ventilator that the client will use at home is different from the one that the client is using in the hospital, the model to be used at home is provided to the hospital at least 1 week before discharge. This allows the family to learn on the appropriate equipment, and it allows the hospital team to evaluate the client's response to this new ventilator. The client and home support team will need to demonstrate, to the satisfaction of the company therapist, at least 48 hours before discharge, appropriate use of the equipment. This includes maintenance and troubleshooting procedures.

At the same time that this training is occurring in the hospital, the home is being readied for the client. At least 1 week before discharge a ventilator is placed in the client's home. A determination is made that all the electrical and structural requirements are met and that support systems are in place. In addition, the telephone, electrical, oil, or gas companies and fire and ambulance departments will be notified by phone and in writing that a ventilator-dependent client will be in this home. The same notification will go to the answering services for the physician, home care agency, and the respiratory equipment company.

On the day of discharge the client must be seen by the pulmonologist. The client is then escorted home by an RN or credentialed respiratory therapy practitioner. All RNs scheduled to care for the client should have extensive experience in ventilator care and current CPR certification. In this therapy the nurse's role as primary care nurse does not really begin until the client is home.

Case Studies

The following case studies represent the three main areas of high-tech home care discussed thus far. The first illustrates a client who received combination therapy that included hyperalimentation, pain control, and chemotherapy. The second client, the most complex case presented, required enteral, hydration, antibiotic, and heparin therapy. The final client requires home ventilator therapy.

Patient 1

Lynn was a 63-year-old woman with primary breast cancer with metastasis to the axilla. She was initially referred to the agency following a radical mastectomy. A Hickman catheter was placed for the provision of hyperalimentation and chemotherapy due to poor peripheral access. Lynn had experienced a 30-pound weight loss over a 3-month period. Her initial orders were for 500 cc of Travesol 8.5% with electrolytes in 500 cc D50W to be infused at 83 cc per hour for 12 hours. On Monday, Wednesday, Friday, and Saturday an additional 500 cc of Intralipid 10% was to be added to the solution to be infused at 125 cc per hour. The hyperalimentation was infused using a HomePro stationary pump. Lynn's chemotherapy orders were for methotrexate 25 mg followed by 5-Fluorouracil 500 mg IV push to be given every other Wednesday. The chemotherapy was curative. Blood work was drawn once weekly to include a CBC, Profile-13, platelet count, and sedimentation rate. Periodic CEA levels were also obtained.

Lynn and her husband both learned the procedures for hooking up and disconnecting the equipment. The procedures were most often performed with Lynn and her husband sharing the individual steps of the procedures. Lynn remained on this regime for 4 months, until December 31, when her hyperalimentation was discontinued. The biweekly chemotherapy, however, continued for another 15 months. Chemotherapy injections were held if her CBC and platelet count fell below acceptable levels.

Lynn's body weight continued to fluctuate during this period as a result of inconsistent eating habits. Her medical history included a history of alcohol (ETOH) abuse. Despite careful teaching and close observation it was suspected that she continued to abuse alcohol. She denied this and was never observed impaired while performing any procedures. It was noted, however, that her husband gradually assumed more responsibility for her care. She was able to gain some weight when she used nutritional supplements, such as Ensure, and did not return to the

extreme weight loss that precipitated her need for hyperalimentation.

Nineteen months after admission to home care a lump was found on Lynn's upper arm. CAT scans confirmed metastasis to bone and lung. Lynn again experienced a precipitous weight loss. Chemotherapy orders were changed to include cytoxin 50 mg daily by mouth, and nutritional supplements were increased. Lynn's condition continued to deteriorate, and she began to experience severe pain from the bone metastasis.

Two years after her admittance to home care Lynn was placed on pain control therapy. A CADD-PCA cassette style pump was used to deliver a continuous infusion of 0.5 mg per hour of morphine. The concentration of the solution was 2 mg/ml in a total volume of 50 ml. Therefore, a 50 ml cassette lasted for a maximum of 8 days with 12 mg (6 ml) delivered daily. Over the next 4 weeks the dosage increased to a total of 1.5 mg/hour.

As the effects of the narcotic caused Lynn to become more sedated, her intake decreased. After 1 month the infusion was transferred to a volume of 2000 cc D51/2NS and placed on a Flo-Gard 6100 pump to provide hydration as well as pain control. Lynn died at home 26 months after being admitted to home care.

Summary: Lynn presented with several problems, all complicated by her ETOH abuse. Although not an ideal situation, it did not preclude her from home IV therapy. To review the areas of assessment discussed earlier: both Lynn and her husband were very interested, committed, and able to learn the therapy. Her therapy was provided easily on a rotating schedule allowing her the freedom to remain active during the daytime. The home chemotherapy weaned her from dependency on her oncolgist and was more convenient. Her improved emotional state contributed to the quality of her last 2 years of life. Because of their familiarity over the 2 years with pumps and equipment, pain control was provided with relative ease and comfort. Lynn lived and died as she wished, at home.

Patient 2

Michael was a 60-year-old man admitted with a primary diagnosis of cancer of the larynx and trachea, complicated by hypothyroidism and sepsis. He was discharged from the hospital on multiple therapies, including enteral feedings via a gastric tube and combination antibiotic, heparin, and hydration therapy via a Hickman catheter. Michael continued to receive inpatient chemotherapy treatments on a monthly basis. This client presented with many complex, interrelated needs.

Michael's hypothyroidism created frequent potentially life-threatening fluctuations in his blood calcium levels. To maintain an even level, his enteral feedings, which contained calcium, his vitamin D supplements, and his intravenous hydration had to be coordinated. Michael was intermittently noncompliant with his regime, either because of gastric distress or depression. Michael's antibiotic therapy was complicated by resistant organisms and superinfections. His general nutritional status contributed to poor healing at his G-tube and tracheal sites.

Michael's wife was a nurse and, therefore, well prepared for learning the techniques of these complex therapies. She, however, had to continue working in order to maintain the insurance benefits that covered this therapy. Nursing service was provided from 8 AM to 4 PM Monday through Friday to allow her to continue to work. Michael's 24-hour regime included

1. Oxacillin 2 g IV piggyback at 8 AM, 12 noon, 4 PM, 8 PM, 12 midnight, and 4 AM
2. Heparin 5000 u IV push at 8 AM, 2 PM, and 8 PM
3. Ensure ½ strength and Enrich ½ strength 800 cc three times daily via the G-tube using the bolus method
4. Blood work was drawn on Monday, Wednesday, and Friday
5. Infusions of ½ strength normal saline were infused in amounts ranging from 1000 to 2000 cc, depending on blood calcium levels

Once monthly Michael was admitted to the hospital to receive an infusion of Cisplatin. This was followed by a ninety-six hour continuous infusion of 5-Fluorouracil 1400 mg given via a CADD 5100 pump. The antibiotic therapy was interrupted during this time period, and enteral feedings were replaced by feedings of plain water to total 3000 cc daily. This reduced his gastric distention, provided adequate hydration, and reduced the risk of aspiration from nausea and vomiting following the Cisplatin. Chemotherapy was interrupted for the bolus injections of heparin.

Four months after admittance to home care Michael was readmitted to the hospital for revision of his laryngectomy. His Hickman catheter was replaced in an attempt to resolve his recurring infections. When he returned home his antibiotic therapy was discontinued. Michael's enteral feedings were changed to Enrich full strength

500 cc with 500 cc water three times daily. The heparin and chemotherapy orders remained unchanged. Blood work was decreased to twice weekly. Michael became more involved in his own therapy and learned to give his own enteral therapy and heparin injections. Hydration was still used on an as-needed basis based on his blood calcium levels. With fewer restrictions from therapy, Michael was able to become more active, taking walks outside and car rides. One month after his second hospitalization private duty nursing was discontinued. Michael's wife, a school nurse, was able to take the summer off.

The following autumn Michael was able to care for himself while his wife worked. This lasted until November when he again began to experience dramatic fluctuations in his calcium levels. A CAT scan confirmed that the tumor had recurred. Private duty nurses were again scheduled to assist in providing hydration therapy. Michael was readmitted to the hospital on Christmas Eve. He was placed on a ventilator in January of the following year. His physician felt that he was not physiologically stable enough to return home on a ventilator.

Summary: Michael's was an extremely complex case with frequent potential for instability. Four things were essential to allow him to participate in home care: His family member's (wife's) ability and commitment, the availability of skilled nurses for both shifts and visits, the availability of appropriate equipment, and most important, a physician who believed it could all be done in the home. The appropriateness of his home care was reevaluated frequently to assure that care was safe, effective, and provided within agency guidelines.

Patient 3

Marion was a 54-year-old woman with COPD and respiratory failure who was ventilator dependent, and she had multiple compression fractures of her dorsal spine. She was discharged to home on an LP 6 ventilator with suction equipment and a PulmoAide. Her husband and mother resided with her and, in conjunction with a nurse during the day, would provide her care.

Marion's blood gases at the time of her discharge were PA(CO_2), 31, PA(O_2),87 and ambient O_2 was 38%. Her ventilator settings were for an assist control of 14 breaths per minute, tidal volume of 700 and 35% O_2. She was bedridden because of multiple fractures of her spine and had multiple decubitus ulcers. Her orders were for PulmoAide treatments four times daily to decrease episodes of pneumonia. In addition, she was to be turned every 2 hours daily through the evening, on a gel mattress to increase her mobilization and circulation and to decrease the incidence of decubitus ulcers.

Her family, primary care nurse, and the day nurse were instructed in the use of the LP 6 ventilator in the hospital before her discharge. Daily the nurse would record the following information on her flow sheet:

- Date and time
- Volume set
- Pressure set
- Actual patient pressure
- Respiratory rate set actual respiratory rate
- Check all settings
- FiO$_2$
- Alarms on
- Temperature of inspired air
- If the circuits were changed and when

Each new nurse was instructed in Marion's care and the functioning of the ventilator by the respiratory therapist of the respiratory company. Because of her constant back pain Marion received narcotic pain control. In addition, she began receiving antidepressant medication 2 months after her discharge for posthospital depression. The combination of the medications depressed her respiratory function. A weaning schedule to decrease her narcotic dependency was begun 3 months after her discharge. This was a slow, difficult process that became cyclical. Her pain was real to her, and decreasing her pain medication made her both angry and depressed. The antidepressants caused mild fluid retention, which affected her respiratory capacity.

Eight months after discharge from the hospital Marion was receiving two shifts of nurses. Her narcotic pain control needs had been reduced by 75% with her pain primarily controlled by nonnarcotic methods. Social work services had been instituted, and a weaning schedule for her antidepressants had begun. Marion remains at home. She has required two short-term hospitalizations in the last 2 years. Her respiratory status continues to decline slowly.

Summary: Ventilator therapy is perhaps the most difficult to plan, evaluate, and institute in the home. The determining factors in Marion's case were her determination to dictate her own life-style, the availability and commitment of her family, and the availability of appropriately trained personnel. Her total dependence, not only on a machine but also on the personnel around her, made home care a challenge.

These case studies have been presented for two reasons. First to provide examples of what is possible outside a hospital setting and second, to provide a basis for the following section. In reading the steps outlined in the following section, the nurse can recreate the planning and implementation involved in each of these cases.

Planning and Implementing High-Tech Therapy

Qualifying the Client. The very first step in dealing with the high-tech client, as discussed earlier in this chapter, is qualifying the client, which involves answering the following questions:

1. Do the client and family accept the proposed therapy? Will they be willing participants?
2. Does the physician accept their decision, and is the physician a willing participant in managing the care of the client?
3. Is the home environment safe for the provision of this therapy?
4. Are the risks, responsibilities, and expected results of the therapy clearly understood by all involved?
5. What type of and how much support personnel will be required, and is that support readily available?
6. What type of equipment is needed, and is it readily available?
7. Is there adequate financial support for the personnel, equipment, drugs, and supplies that are required?

Once these have been evaluated to the agency's satisfaction the client can be accepted into the program. The success of high-tech home care is based on sound preliminary assessment and planning started in the hospital, well before the date of discharge.

Once the client is qualified for home care, the primary nurse, in conjunction with the hospital and equipment company, must perform discharge planning. The ease of completing this process will depend on the company and hospital dealt with. In high-tech care the home care nurse must maintain her position as primary coordinator of discharge plans. In reality this is often difficult. Hospital discharge planners and coordinators from equipment and pharmaceutical companies will also view themselves in this role, but, once the client is home, full responsibility will revert to the home health agency. It is essential that the nurse is directly involved in all the *pre*discharge decisions and coordination of all events from hospital to home to ensure a safe and controlled transition.

Pre-discharge planning from the hospital includes the following steps.

1. Preparing the home environment to receive the client

2. Ordering and confirming the setup of all equipment
3. Ordering and confirming delivery of all medications and supplies
4. Establishing the teaching plans and time frame and completing preparations to accomplish them. This includes confirming that predischarge teaching has been completed and that personnel are scheduled for any teaching that will be done in the home
5. Establishing the need for support personnel and the scheduling of that personnel
6. Ensuring that emergency plans are in place
7. Establishing a confirmed discharge date and time
8. Planning for appropriate transportation from hospital to home with escort personnel as needed

Preparation of the home environment includes setup of the sick room, including a hospital bed, commode, and ambulation equipment. When a ventilator or stationary intravenous or enteral pump is being used, these also should be set up and their functioning checked. Any necessary modifications to the plan can be identified at this time. For example, since ambulation was difficult for Michael, two stationary intravenous pumps were ordered for him. This allowed him the freedom of spending his days downstairs and evenings upstairs. The change of environment was essential for his mental and emotional well-being.

Ordering equipment, supplies, and medications for these complex therapies becomes very difficult when many different vendors are involved. When ordering equipment, supplies, and medications it is extremely helpful to have one vendor available to provide most or all of the client's supplies. For example, Michael's vendor was able to supply all his equipment, medications, enteral and intravenous solutions, and his tracheostomy care supplies. The time of delivery was set for 12 to 24 hours before discharge to allow review of the order for discrepancies and to enable last minute changes, such as the extra pump. Remember, based on stability and shelf life, some medications may require a second delivery closer to the time of the client's discharge from the hospital.

The decision to begin teaching before discharge or to wait until the client is home depends on several factors. The first factor is **hospital policy regarding patient contact** by someone not employed by the hospital or a family member. It is well within the hospital's legal rights to restrict access to the patient and his or her clinical record. A second factor is the **teaching environment**. The client can often be complacent in the hospital and, as a result, be a poor learner. The reality of his actually performing the procedures may only become real to him at home.

Liability is a third factor that restricts the nurse as an agent of the agency teaching or performing any procedures for which the hospital may be liable. For example, if while the home care nurse is teaching the heparin flush procedure to a client in the hospital an air embolus occurs, the question of which is liable, the agency or hospital, arises. The final factor is whether the client can safely be discharged from the hospital *without prior teaching*. In the case of home ventilator therapy it is obvious that the client must be instructed in the hospital. With less complicated therapies, such as enteral or antibiotic therapy, teaching can begin at home as long as support personnel are available at the time of each procedure until the client and family are independent.

The need for support personnel must be assessed and a schedule developed before hospital discharge. For example, Michael required a registered nurse for a full shift, whereas Lynn needed only two visits daily, at the times of her procedures. It is important that the support personnel's activities be reviewed to assure they have the proper skills.

Anticipation of and preparation for emergencies is best done at the time agency policies and protocols are established. Unexpected events can have a far more devastating effect on the high-tech client. For example, support personnel can be delayed or unable to work, equipment can malfunction, power outages can occur rendering equipment unusable, or the client may panic while performing a procedure.

Finally, coordinating the date and time of discharge is important. A quick phone call to the hospital on the morning of discharge is recommended. Changes can occur overnight in the client's condition, and communication of a change in discharge plans may not occur in time. To plan for transportation from hospital to home, contact the hospital discharge planner as this is often within the scope of their responsibilities. The discharge planner will need to know any special requirements, such as ventilator or intravenous equipment, that will be needed during transport.

The Day of Discharge. Even the most well planned discharge day can be chaotic. Plan to be at the client's home before he or she arrives. Once the client has arrived, take charge and get the client settled first. Do not plan to do any extensive teaching at this time. The high-tech patient is usually more ill and, therefore, more tired. The sight of the equipment in the home may be too overwhelming. A fatigued, anxious client is a poor learner.

Provide the client and family with a general overview of the next 24 to 48 hours. Guide them step by step through the expected events. For example,

"Mrs. Jones, I am here now to begin your intravenous therapy. I will do the procedure today and ask you to watch. Tomorrow I will actually begin to teach you. I will stay with you now to show you what to do if any alarms ring or problems arise. Here are our phone numbers, where you can reach a nurse any time of the day or night. Jane will be here at 8 PM tonight to disconnect you from the pump. I will return at 8 AM tomorrow morning to begin teaching you the hookup procedure that you will be performing. After that there will be a nurse here each day at 8 AM and 8 PM until you are completely comfortable with the procedure and can perform it without assistance."

The first 48 to 72 hours at home are critical. To make the transition from the hospital to home the client must feel that support is readily and rapidly available. Appendix 6 is an example of an emergency phone list for the client. Included on the emergency list should be the client's therapy so that the information is readily available at the time of an emergency. The list provides assurance to the caregiver and can save precious minutes in an emergency.

A sample of client instructions can be obtained from any national or local pharmaceutical company providing home intravenous therapy. Instructions can be developed for each type of therapy and left in a prominent place in the home. Easily understood language and clear, concise, and abbreviated instructions should be used. The client should be provided with a loose-leaf style home chart in which all instructions, care plans, and clinical notes can be kept. A standard format should be established and maintained so that all personnel can readily locate needed information.

Once the client has been settled at home, equipment checked, therapy started, and questions answered the initial visit is completed. The nurse should follow the visit with a phone call 1 to 3 hours afterward; this assures the family that the nurse really is just a phone call away. The nurse should also contact any support personnel to update them to the client's condition, review what was taught, and relay any concerns or complaints expressed by the client. The initial visit can often take 2 to 4 hours, and sufficient time should be allowed to avoid being rushed.

Clinical Management

The primary nurse's role in the ongoing clinical management of the client includes the following: teaching, ongoing evaluation of the client and therapy, maintenance of adequate documentation, and acting as liaison between the client, family, physician, agency personnel, and drug and equipment vendors. Each of these will be examined separately.

Teaching High-Tech Care. Teaching high-tech home care can be both rewarding and frustrating. Unlike less acute home care, very complex material must be learned rapidly and thoroughly by the client. It is far more difficult to teach a client to administer chemotherapy by means of a central catheter than it is to teach the basics of a low-salt diet. The principles delineated in chapter 4, particularly Bloom's three learning domains, should be clearly understood and utilized as the basis for any teaching.

First it is important to understand those characteristics that make teaching high-tech care different from teaching general home care topics. These are

1. The equipment and procedures taught are often highly technical.
2. Very broad principles and theories, such as aseptic technique, form the basis of the technical procedures. These principles must be taught in a concise format without sacrificing safety.
3. The amount of information to be learned is vast. It must be reduced to a concise, logical, and clear package of information that the client can assimilate rapidly and thoroughly.
4. Troubleshooting and emergency procedures must be taught frequently before important underlying concepts can be learned and understood by the client.
5. The patient or caregiver must possess excellent functional ability and manual dexterity to perform the actual tasks.
6. The procedures, equipment, and therapies themselves are often new to the home care nurse.

By understanding the cognitive domain and these six characteristics of high-tech home care and how they relate an effective teaching plan can be prepared and implemented.

The first domain, the cognitive domain, encompasses these learning skills. In order for the client to be left unattended with a functioning pump he or she must know the mechanical parts of the pump and how to use them (e.g., the rate/dose or on/off buttons) (knowledge). To perform the "programming procedure" dosage for the pump the client must know the rate and dose of his medication or solution and how the rate and dose are programmed into the pump (comprehension). The client must actually set the pump to deliver his or her medication at the prescribed rate and dose (application). If the "high pressure" alarm sounds, the client must know this means there is a blockage in the tubing (analysis), how to eliminate the blockage (synthesis), how to reset the pump and assess for the patency of the line following this procedure (evaluation). Teaching high-tech care is not simply a matter of demonstrating a series of steps and explaining a few dos and don'ts.

Examples of Teaching. The following exercises will illustrate the complexities of the subject matter to be taught by the home care nurse.

1. To begin, the nurse should list each step of the procedure she is planning to teach. The underlying principles the client needs to understand to be able to perform that task should be written in parentheses. For example, the procedure to draw up a syringe of heparin flush would be
   a. Gather supplies (identify technical names)
   b. Wash hands (aseptic technique)
   c. Open syringe package (aseptic technique)
   d. Draw air into syringe (air pressure/fluid displacement)
   e. Clean top of vial (aseptic technique)
   f. Insert needle into vial (aseptic technique)
   g. Inject air into vial and withdraw heparin (air pressure/fluid displacement)
   h. Withdraw 3 cc of heparin (medication dosage)
   i. Expel air bubbles from syringe (air embolus)
   j. Replace syringe needle cap (aseptic technique)
2. Now this same exercise with the entire antibiotic procedure, including preparation, administration, and discontinuance of the dose via a peripheral heparin lock, should be performed. The nurse must remember to include programming and troubleshooting the pump and equipment and assessing the patency of the intravenous line in this exercise.
   The following activities should not be overlooked: (1) checking the label for client name, dose, and solution; (2) checking the solution for discoloration and sediment; and (3) proper disposal of the needles, syringes, and supplies. These and other steps are often overlooked. They are steps that the nurse herself no longer practices or are so basic that they are overlooked. Teaching high-tech care can be a *reeducation* for the teaching nurse at the same time that it is an *education* for the client.
3. The lists must then be broken down into teaching units. The nurse can sit down with a coworker and actually teach one section including any demonstrations and return demonstrations. How long did it take to teach the section? Did the nurse find herself straying outside the prescribed contents of that section to make the material more understandable? Was there too little (or too much) information to absorb in one sitting? These exercises can reveal how tedious, time consuming, and sometimes confusing teaching high-tech material to a lay person can be.

The second domain, the affective domain, is equally important to teaching high-tech home care. The client or caregiver's involvement and commitment to learning the material may be different in the hospital than in the home. High-tech therapies can be frightening and overwhelming. Movement through the four affective levels is often far slower than when learning less complicated procedures, and the acuity of the client's condition can impair learning and create backslides to lower levels of comprehension.

The final domain, the psychomotor domain, is frequently overlooked. Many of the tasks that must be performed require a high level of manual dexterity. To understand this concept better, the nurse can review what physical abilities (manual dexterity) are required to perform the heparin flush procedure. Notice how the end of the heparin lock must be held free from contamination in one hand, while the syringe needle is uncapped with the other hand, without contaminating either the needle or injection port. Does the new staff nurse remember how long it took to attain the manual dexterity and confidence to perform this task? Often the actual physical process involved in performing these intricate tasks can be more frustrating than learning the technical terms and procedures. By using pictorial and video aids and actual demonstration the nurse can help the client visualize what must be done. Consistency in teaching is paramount to reducing anxiety. Working with unfamiliar equipment can feel less threatening if the client learns only *one* way to handle the materials. To understand the lay person's perspective better the nurse could have someone teach her how to use chopsticks. Do the chopsticks feel awkward? Is it difficult to translate the instructions into actions? The nurse may find herself a lay person in regard to this learning material just as her client might to the technical material presented.

As discussed earlier, preparation and organization will assure the best possible outcome when teaching high-tech material. Thorough development of care plans and utilization of checklists and outlines will prepare the nurse to teach competently and confidently, and these tools will serve as the basis for accurate and complete documentation, including the principles and procedures taught and the learner's response to the material. Appendix 7 is an example of a teaching checklist that can be used as a tool and as legal confirmation that teaching has been completed.

Breaking material down to separate related components makes the task easier. For example, Lynn's (patient 1) teaching was divided into three teaching topics, (1) her Hickman catheter and its care; (2) her chemotherapy and hyperalimentation and their effects and side effects; and (3) the equipment and its operation. Another factor that the nurse must consider is a decision must also be made how much detailed technical material will be included. Some learners benefit from a more in-depth explanation while that same information may frighten or confuse another. It is important to tie related information together for the client. For instance, when teaching aseptic technique, the nurse must teach that it is important to observe aseptic technique when spiking the bag as well as when attaching the needle. All of these elements are part of the same "system," and bacteria in one area can cause the same harm that bacteria in another area can.

Two tools for teaching high-tech home care are found in client-oriented instructional material and in Standard High Tech care plans (see Appendix 8). The nurse's teaching material must be clear, concise, and written in understandable language. Vendors often have teaching materials that can be adapted to the home care nurse's needs. If several vendors with many different types of equipment are to be used by the client, a teaching tool that is generic and includes blank fill-in spaces to identify the particulars of each piece of equipment is best.

Prewritten care plans serve a twofold purpose; they assure consistent care based on agency policies and procedures, and they serve as references for caregivers and agency personnel. Prewritten care plans guarantee that all procedures and information will be addressed consistently from client to client. Care plans can be completed for specific disease processes, procedures, therapies or nursing diagnoses. Only those that pertain to a specific client are chosen. A comprehensive care plan that ties the prewritten plans together can be written tailored to each client.

The goal for the high-tech patient is to understand the basic principles of how the equipment functions and the interactions between the medications and the client's body. He or she must understand why procedures must be performed *exactly* as they are taught. The goal for the nurse-teacher is to make the client safely independent in his or her procedures with a clear understanding of what is abnormal and what to do when a problem develops. As professionals there are often shortcuts in technique that nurses use in the client's presence. It is important to be aware of these and to caution the client *never* to try what the nurse is doing. The client must have a clear understanding of the following:

1. **When** to call the nurse or the physician
2. What **never** to do
3. What **always** to do

For example, Lynn could not grasp the concept of an air embolus. To ensure safety she was taught to *always* clamp the Hickman line whenever that alarm sounded on her pump. She was also instructed *never* to open the internal clamp on the pump until she had called the on-call nurse.

The teacher is as critical to the teaching process as are the learner and the material. Regardless of previous experience the high-tech teacher will continually be faced with having to supplement her knowledge base with new information. As the name makes clear, high-tech care is very technical, with rapid new developments. Bridging these knowledge gaps on an ongoing basis is essential to allow the teacher to teach confidently and competently. The nurse's personal attitudes and values also affect the effectiveness of your teaching. Pain control, chemotherapy, and ventilator therapy can be controversial therapies, especially when used with terminal clients. The cost, complexity, and even the goals of many therapies can conflict with the nurse's personal values and beliefs. The nurse must examine how she feels about the proposed plan of care before teaching a client. It is better to relinquish responsibility to another professional than to compromise the client's care and learning.

Much of the nursing care in high-tech home care can be considered troubleshooting. Because of the complexity of the therapies, much of the nurse's time will be spent addressing such issues as reprogramming pumps, adjusting dosage schedules, and reviewing procedures. The client, after teaching will have a rudimentary knowledge of the pump or ventilator, their alarms and what to do when they sound, and the nurse will frequently find herself on the other end of the phone with a "problem with a pump" or a question about a procedure. Unlike less acute care, the need is usually of an urgent nature and cannot wait until a home visit can be arranged. These problems cannot be avoided, but they can be anticipated.

Written instructional material pertaining to each hi-tech client's care is essential. Each manufacturer has easy-to-read guides for clients in addition to their technical manuals. The agency should compile, in a concise manner, essential information on the pumps, medications, accompanying supplies and equipment that the nurse uses, with space to write in further comments. This information in a book format can be supplied to the office and to the on-call nurses. It saves precious minutes when the pump has malfunctioned or when reprogramming is required. The nurse will, through experience, discover what other information is frequently needed about the various therapies, supplies, and equipment. The best resources for this kind of information are the people that work with the equipment frequently, such as the nurses, pharmacists, and therapists in the vendor companies.

Documentation of High-Tech Home Care. Documentation is of primary importance in high-tech care. To assure that it is complete one or both of the following methods should be employed. One method is provided in Appendix 9, the clinical flow sheet. This can be supplemented by flow sheets for lab work (see Appendix 10) or flow sheets for recording daily weight, temperature, urine sugar, and acetones for the client on hyperalimentation. These are completed by a note expanding on any identified problems. A second method is a documentation outline. This serves as a guideline for each professional of the parameters that must be addressed in each note. Preferably a combination of both methods will assure that nothing is assumed, overlooked, or omitted in the documentation.

Documentation Outlines. The following are examples of documentation outlines to be documented in each clinical note. These are not a complete listing but rather guidelines specific to the therapies. These should be tailored to the specific client (e.g., describing the wound) and by information specifically required by your agency.

ENTERAL THERAPY

1. Date and time of visit
2. Solution, volume, rate, and method of delivery (bolus or drip)
3. Placement of feeding tube and how evaluated
4. The client's tolerance of the feeding since the last visit
5. Physical assessment, including weight and periodic temperatures, fluid and electrolyte balances (lab values)

INTRAVENOUS THERAPY

1. Date and time of visit
2. Administration site appearance (peripheral or central line)
3. Method of site change or accessing and dressing change technique
4. Name, dose, rate, and method of administration of all medications or solutions administered
5. Name of pump and pump settings
6. Topics taught and client response, including return demonstration (e.g., hookup or disconnect procedure). Make specific reference to teaching tools (e.g., "Hookup procedure taught according to agency protocols as found in client care plan")

VENTILATOR THERAPY

1. Date and time of visit
2. Ventilator settings and readings at time of visit
3. Physical assessment, including heart and lung sounds
4. Summary of respiratory therapy notes since last visit

One of the responsibilities of the primary nurse is the ongoing evaluation of the client and his or her therapy. Due to the severity of the client's condition,

physical assessments are usually more involved and more frequent. The clinical flow sheet (Appendix 9) for the high-tech client provides an overview of the client's physical assessment and client complaints at a glance. This type of a flow sheet allows the nurse to sort rapidly through a volume of information. For example, a pattern was readily visible when reviewing Michael's flow sheet. A correlation could be made between his intake and his calcium levels.

The contents of the nurse's documentation will be affected by state licensure laws, each state's nurse practice act, federal requirements, insurance coverage requirements, and agency policies and procedures. An outline or flowsheet, or both, should be used to ensure that all the information required is in each and every clinical note.

Resources are readily available. Large pharmaceutical companies have teaching materials, drug information, pump programming information, and, often, research materials on new therapies. There are computer programs that can tap research hospitals for chemotherapy protocols. The pharmacists in the pharmaceutical companies can provide much information about the stability, shelf life, and compatibility of medications and solutions. They can also assist in deciding which pump to use. The nurse representatives in these same companies can provide much information about supplies and equipment, such as peripheral intravenous equipment. The additional resources for this book will also provide other resources for information about such topics as chemotherapy, intravenous therapy, hyperalimentation, and pain control.

One of the prime objectives of high-tech home care is to provide continuity and quality of care. Following the steps outlined in this section will provide the tools to do this. First, make a sound educated decision to admit a client for high-tech home care. Second, perform thorough predischarge planning. Third, provide only qualified personnel and ensure that the client is meticulously taught and safely cared for. Fourth, make sure that all the documentation is complete and precise. Finally, anticipate and plan for disruptions and problems by having and providing resource materials and contingency plans. Although actually doing all these things may not fall within the home care nurse's job description, they must all be in place for the client to receive quality care with continuity.

Discharging a Client. When it comes time to discharge a client from high-tech home care, the entire case must be reviewed carefully. The nurse's discharge summary and plan will need to be more detailed than a summary for a less acutely ill client. It will need to include the outcome of the therapy and whether it was "successful." Coverage guidelines should be reviewed before writing about the therapy's outcome. Many variables change with the high-tech patient. The *goal* of therapy is often the determinant of insurance coverage, and a misinterpreted discharge summary can have an adverse effect on the coverage provided. Documentation must also be reviewed to make sure it is complete. Insurance companies are increasingly requiring complete copies of nurse's notes and physician's orders. If the photocopying is a clerical duty it is the nurse's responsibility to make sure that the information is correct before it is sent to the insurance provider. Again, poor documentation can have an adverse effect on coverage. What might have appeared adequate on the day it was written may not look as complete in review.

Policies and Nursing Procedures

Policies and procedures form the foundation for any well-run nursing program. This is not to suggest that it is the primary nurse's responsibility to develop them, however, she will function within them. The policies and procedures will restrict and protect the home care nurse. Good resources for developing these are the pharmaceutical and equipment vendors with whom the nurse deals. They have greater resources of information and have already developed sound policies and procedures. When dealing with a new or established company the nurse should ask to review their policies. The policies can be compared with the nurse's own or incorporated into a new program, if the nurse is developing it for a new therapy. This will allow the nurse to assess whether the vendor company to be dealt with is a reputable one.

Policies and procedures protect the nurse by providing a basis from which to work. When they are incorporated into the home care nurse's daily functions and into documentation there is no guess work as to the quality of the care provided. When problems arise, care that was provided based on sound policies and procedures protects both the nurse and the agency from liability. Another benefit is that policies protect the nurse in case she is asked to provide unorthodox or unsafe care.

Policies and procedures can also be restrictive. Each procedure will be performed according to the agency's policies, and those policies that are outdated by current standard can be cumbersome and, at times, costly. For example, intravenous restart kits are fairly standard today and usually are cost-effective. If the agency's policies call for different solutions or supplies than those contained in the kit, ordering custom kits or ordering each item separately may be more costly to the agency or to the client. The nurse should review policies and procedures before

they are put into effect or are renewed. The nurse and client are the ones most directly affected by them.

Summary

High-tech home care is becoming an integral part of the health care system of the present and future. It is complex, challenging, and exciting. The decision to provide high-tech care for any client is based on a thorough assessment of several critical factors. These include (1) client, family, and physician commitment and involvement; (2) safety factors, including the home environment, the mental, emotional, and physical status of the client and family; (3) availability of equipment and personnel; and (4) sufficient financial resources. This assessment must be completed and evaluated before high-tech home care is considered further.

When high-tech home care is chosen as an option, careful planning must be done to ensure safe, consistent, quality care. Predischarge planning is done in the weeks and days before the client's actual discharge from the hospital. It is imperative that the designated home care professional be intimately involved in all stages of the predischarge and discharge plans. The goal is to ensure a safe transition from hospital to home, and once home, a safe course of therapy. The day of discharge is often the most critical. Sufficient time and personnel must be scheduled to cover both anticipated and unanticipated client needs.

Teaching is of equal importance to the assessment and discharge planning responsibilities in high-tech home care. There are several important characteristics that distinguish high-tech teaching. The basis, however, is the same for all home care teaching, and thorough planning will ensure successful learning. The nurse-teacher must continually keep abreast of developments in equipment, supplies, and the various therapies in order to provide accurate instruction. Resources for instruction are readily available from pharmacists, pharmaceutical and medical supply companies, and from hospitals.

Hi-tech home care is an exciting and rewarding field. It is complex and often frustrating, but with thorough planning it can be extremely successful.

Clinical management of the client is more complex in high-tech home care than it is for most general home care. The nurse must have or develop the necessary assessment and technical skills to manage the client's various needs. Client visits are generally more frequent and of greater length than for less acute care. Documentation must be explicit and must consistently include all information that is deemed necessary, as explained in this chapter. The goal of clinical management is to provide acute care in the home setting in a safe, efficient, and effective manner, and the client or caregiver must become independent in all aspects of care. The policies and procedures that govern the home care nurse's actions must be reviewed on a regular basis for appropriateness. All care must adhere strictly to these policies and procedures to ensure client safety and protect agency personnel from undue legal liability.

HIGH-TECH PEDIATRIC HOME CARE

Caring for children in their home was pioneered by community health nurses in the United States in the late 1800s. In the past several years, caring for severely ill children has been moved from the hospital to home for various reasons that will be discussed in this section. With this movement, performing more high-technology procedures in the home geared for the pediatric population has also increased significantly in the past few years, with children cared for on ventilators, short-and long-term intravenous therapy as well as caring for the terminally ill child at home.

In this section, high-tech pediatric home care and major situations encountered by the home care nurse related to caring for ill children in the home will be discussed. An overview of the role and function of the home care nurse relating to pediatric clients will be discussed, with guidelines for specific types of clients presented. Generic care plans for various client situations are found in Appendix 11 and will assist the home care nurse in planning individualized care for children and their families.

Factors Contributing to the Need for High-Tech Pediatric Home Care

There are four major factors contributing to the need for high-tech pediatric home care. There are approximately 10 million children in the United States who are considered chronically ill. The numbers of these children has increased steadily over the past two decades to the current level due to the tremendous advances in medical and surgical technologies. Premature and low-birth-weight infants, who previously would have died from severe respiratory problems, are now surviving. These infants, however, are often left with bronchopulmonary dysplasia, apnea, and tracheal stenosis.

Surgical advances have meant that children with congenital defects, such as heart disease and spina bifida, are surviving, but also may be left with ongoing deficits. Children with illnesses acquired later in childhood are also reaping the benefits of advanced technology. Children with cancer, asthma, cystic fibrosis, diabetes, muscular dystrophy, cerebral palsy,

infections, and injuries are now living full and productive lives into adulthood.

The second major factor contributing to the increase in pediatric home care is advanced equipment technology, which allows more high-risk and chronically ill children to be cared for at home. Availability and ease in use of equipment, such as ventilators, infusion pumps, monitors, suction machines, phototherapy lights, and nebulizers have allowed children to receive tracheostomy care, dialysis, enteral and parenteral nutrition, intravenous antibiotics, and respiratory therapy in the comfort of their homes.

The cost-effectiveness of pediatric home care, as compared with hospital care, is an important third factor contributing to the use of pediatric home care. Although the general cost-effectiveness of pediatric home care can be supported by several studies, it cannot be applied in all cases (Cabin, 1985). Macmarik and Thompson (1986) found that the average cost of caring for a ventilator-dependent child at home is 87% less than in a hospital setting. Other studies have shown that home care costs of caring for children with other high-tech needs are about 70% less than hospital costs (Goldberg, Faure, Vaughn, Sharski, & Seleny, 1984), and it appears that over time the cost of home care declines. The longer the child is home and the more the child's health improves, the overall plan becomes simplified and other family members participate in the care plan. Third party payors are beginning to recognize these cost savings and are looking at improving benefits for home care coverage, especially to prevent rehospitalization.

The final and most significant factor for the increase is the benefit of home care to the child. A child's development in the hospital tends to regress, whereas the child's development at home tends to advance, despite the presence of a chronic, debilitating illness. Normal interactions with parents and siblings have a positive effect on the physical, emotional, and social well-being of ill children. The most successful pediatric home care plans are those that combine optimal medical technology and support with the benefits of normal family relationships to promote growth and development in ill children.

Discharge Planning

Initial Planning. Planning for the unique and individual home care needs of the ill child presents many challenges but also offers the satisfaction of giving the child and family the opportunity to continue living in a cohesive family unit. A commitment to normalizing the life of the child while providing adequate medical, nursing, and emotional support to the family is the primary goal in bringing the ill child home.

Planning and coordination of home care services must be a team effort. The primary physician, nurse, social worker, and home care agency must all work together to provide the best continuity and quality of care possible. Initial planning involves researching the family's health insurance coverage. If there is a lack of adequate reimbursement for home care, any type of home care plan, no matter how basic, becomes problematic.

Funding. Each state has an individual Medicaid policy, which is specific regarding income eligibility, services, and equipment covered. This is described in detail in Chapter 1. Private insurance companies and health maintenance organizations (HMOs) have greatly varying policies for home care. It is often possible to negotiate with insurance companies and other payment sources by documenting that the cost of home care would be considerably less expensive than hospital care. Other sources of funding are local community organizations and private foundations or the State Crippled Children's Program (Ahmann, 1986).

Discharge Assessment. The next phase of discharge planning is assessment of the child's and family's needs, determining the nursing care plan and setting up a working relationship between the family and health professionals. Family assessment includes looking at the family's understanding of the diagnosis, prognosis, and actual care required. What is the family's attitude toward the child's illness? Are parents able to demonstrate adequate responsibility? Is the physical environment of the home conducive to home care?

Regular, predischarge conferences assist in communicating needs, setting goals, and determining readiness for discharge. To enhance continuity of care, the conferences should include all appropriate hospital and home care personnel. Parents should be involved also, since they need to become increasingly comfortable with child advocacy and identifying their own learning needs, as well as become comfortable with the total home care plan.

Implementing the Home Care Plan. Implementation of the home care plan involves parent and professional education, the ordering of equipment, and making appropriate referrals for community services. Parent or caregiver teaching stresses the details of routine and potential emergency care. Discussion, written materials, and demonstration by the nurse are the usual techniques. Return demonstration of materials learned is essential and will provide evidence of confidence and competence. Caregivers should be al-

lowed extended periods of time when they are given total responsibility for the child's care in the hospital while having easy access to professional support.

Home care nurses and other personnel who will be providing services in the home also need to be confident and comfortable with the different aspects of the child's care. They too, must have the opportunity to become familiar with the child's care before discharge from the hospital. Parents should never be responsible for training professional home care personnel.

Selection of an appropriate equipment vendor is imperative to providing a positive home care experience for the family. According to Hartsell and Ward (1985) the following are important criteria to consider for choosing an equipment vendor.

1. 24-hour availability
2. Home visits to provide follow-up instruction and support
3. Pediatric experience and equipment
4. Ability to service and replace equipment
5. Provision of written instructions on operation and maintenance of equipment

Referrals to community services may include not only the local home health agency but also private duty home care nursing agencies, parent–infant education programs, or parent support groups. Referrals should be made well before the anticipated date of discharge to avoid gaps in service. Notifying home care early on allows the home care nurse ample time to become familiar with the care, visit the child while hospitalized, and make a predischarge home visit, if necessary. Teaching checklists and a written plan of care should be provided for the home care nurse from the institution. Other therapeutic needs the child may have might indicate physical, occupational, speech, and respiratory therapy referrals. Referrals for professional respite care may be needed as well, based on the family's need for extended hours of nursing care. Several agencies may need to be involved to provide adequate coverage.

Role of the Home Health Agency

It is important that the home health agency engaged have a formal pediatric home care program in operation, since home care nursing holds a key case management function in caring for a child in the home. Ideally, the program should have a pediatric clinical nurse specialist and trained pediatric home care nurses. The pediatric clinical nurse specialist takes responsibility for staff education, case consultation, and quality assurance activities. The agency should have written policies and procedures regarding care of children in the home.

A standard pediatric assessment form should be used in an agency to document each pediatric home visit. This pediatric assessment form includes a prenatal history, significant health history of the child including a review of systems, and information regarding nutrition, safety, development, and social information.

The nurse as case manager, is responsible for performing accurate assessments, teaching, documentation, and an update of the care plan. The nurse is in a key position to provide ongoing communication with the physician and other health care personnel on the child's health status. The physician depends on the nurse's assessments to manage and prescribe home treatments or medications.

The needs of ill children at home may be quite complex and involve many different types of personnel. The home care nurse, physician, physical therapist, occupational therapist, speech therapist, nutritionist, social worker, home health aide, a teacher, and private duty nurse must all function as a team. If the personnel involved do not all work for the same agency there needs to be an even greater effort made at communication and coordination. The nurse may find it beneficial to call team meetings periodically to facilitate the coordination and continuity of care.

Guidelines for Specific Types of High-Tech Pediatric Home Care Clients

The following material outlines the home care nursing care needed by children with various problems. Generic care plans that can be used with these clients can be found in Appendix 11 and should be used by the home care nurse to become familiar with the care needed for this unique group of clients.

Respiratory Problems. Home care for the child with a respiratory problem may involve one or more of the following: apnea monitor, oxygen therapy, tracheostomy, or ventilator.

Home Apnea Monitoring. Children requiring the use of apnea monitors fall into three major categories: (1) premature infants with apnea, (2) those who have experienced or are at risk for experiencing a life-threatening event, and (3) at high risk for sudden infant death syndrome (SIDS).

Guidelines for home infant apnea monitoring are not standardized, but there are general indications for monitoring. Documented apnea lasting more than 20 seconds, or an apneic episode associated with cyanosis are the most common indicators for monitor use. Monitors are discontinued when an infant has been without apnea for 6–8 weeks. If an infant is on oxygen or medications, the monitor is usually contin-

ued 6 to 8 weeks beyond the time when all therapy has been discontinued. Home monitoring for most infants is discontinued prior to one year of age. Infants and children with chronic respiratory conditions, for example, a tracheostomy, will require monitoring indefinitely since these children remain at high risk for fatal apnea (Klijanowicz, 1985).

Before hospital discharge, teaching should begin, and reinforcement should be provided on the follow-up home visits after discharge. Topics to be covered are normal infant breathing patterns for sleep and awake states, definition of apnea as it affects the infant, situations likely to provoke apnea, appropriate response to apnea, infant cardiopulmonary resuscitation (CPR), and the operation of the monitor. The family's ability to tolerate the increased stress of home infant monitoring must be assessed and the nurse may make a referral to a support group that could be useful to the family. Home care services for the child on an apnea monitor should include

1. Home nursing visits to assess the infant's cardiopulmonary status, review teaching, and assess the parents' abilities and stresses
2. Home visits from the monitor supplier to review monitor operation and to check home safety

Home Oxygen Therapy. Children with chronic pulmonary and cardiac conditions, which result in chronic hypoxia, are typical candidates for the use of home oxygen therapy. These children fall into two categories. The first category consists of the children who have serious cardiopulmonary dysfunction but have the potential to recover, for example, infants with bronchopulmonary dysplasia. Goals for these children are to wean the child from oxygen, prevent respiratory infections, control cor pulmonale, and enhance growth and development.

The second category of children needing oxygen therapy are those who have an end-stage disease (e.g., cystic fibrosis) that is stable or progressing. Nursing goals with these children are to promote comfort and quality of life for as long as possible.

The type of oxygen delivery varies with the age and diagnosis of the child and equipment availability. Infants will most likely use a nasal cannula or hood, whereas an older child may benefit more from a face mask. Home care services for the child receiving oxygen therapy should include

1. Home care nursing visits to assess the child's cardiopulmonary and nutritional status, assess if oxygen delivery is appropriate and equipment is being used correctly, review teaching, especially safety precautions, CPR, and evaluate the infant's respiratory status

2. Home visits from the oxygen supplier to replace the supply on a regular basis. The oxygen company should have a backup supply available in case of equipment malfunction or oxygen depletion

Home Tracheostomy Care. Common reasons for tracheostomies in children are airway obstruction and inability to raise secretions. The causes for airway obstruction may be central nervous system vocal cord paralysis, subglottic web, cystic hygroma, subglottic hemangioma, or subglottic stenosis. Inability to raise secretions may be caused by bronchopulmonary dysplasia, cystic fibrosis, pneumonia, or diaphragm dysfunction.

Before hospital discharge, the home care nurse should be informed about what the parents have been taught so that appropriate plans for teaching and home follow-up can be made by the primary caregiver in the hospital. A predischarge home visit may be helpful if assessment of the home environment is needed. Home care services for the child with a tracheostomy include

1. Home care nursing visits to assess the child's respiratory status, quality of secretions, appropriateness of equipment and supplies, parents' competence in all aspects of tracheostomy care, which includes suctioning, changing tubes, CPR, and emergency procedures
2. Home visits from equipment vendor for instruction and servicing of equipment

Home Ventilator Care. The reasons for using mechanical ventilation in children range from congenital to acquired conditions involving cardiopulmonary, neuron, skeletal or central nervous control of breathing. Home care may not be appropriate for all children who are ventilator dependent. Factors that must be considered before beginning discharge planning for these children are stability of the disease process, motivation of the family to learn the necessary care, adaptability of the home environment, and availability of a community support system (Ahmann, 1986).

As previously mentioned, the home care nurse should be informed of all teaching done in the hospital and the need for reinforcement once the child is home. Extensive education with all caregivers is essential in suctioning, tracheostomy care, operation and cleaning of equipment, identifying signs of respiratory distress, and performing CPR. Home care services for the ventilator-dependent child include

1. Home care nursing visits to assess the child's clinical status, teach and reinforce skills of caregivers, implementation of infection control measures, assess appropriateness of equipment and supplies

2. Respiratory therapy to assess the functioning and effectiveness of oxygen administration and ventilation and perform oxygenation studies
3. Home visits from equipment vendor to teach operation and maintenance of ventilator and oxygen administration and assess safety of home environment

Gastrointestinal Problems

Tube Feedings. Home care for the child with a gastrointestinal or nutritional problem will usually involve tube feedings or colostomy care. Tube feedings become necessary when a child cannot accept adequate oral feedings. Common reasons include prematurity, cardiopulmonary conditions, and gastroesophageal reflux. Tube feedings may compromise all or part of the child's total nutritional requirements, depending on the child's tolerance of the procedure and physical condition.

Methods of tube feedings are nasogastric (NG), gastrostomy (G), nasojejunal, and jejunostomy. Nasogastric or G tube feedings may be done as a bolus or over a long period of time using a feeding pump. A feeding pump is almost always used with jejunal feedings.

Before the hospital discharge, the family must demonstrate complete responsibility for feeding over a 24-hour period. The home care nurse should be aware of all teaching done, the family's demonstrated abilities, and all equipment and supplies needed. Home care services for the child receiving tube feedings include

1. Home care nursing visits to teach and assess tube feeding techniques, positioning of child, positioning of tube, aspiration precautions, skin care, and growth and development
2. Home visits from equipment vendor to teach operation and maintenance of feeding pump
3. When oral feedings are instituted it may be helpful to consult a speech therapist to assist in developing a feeding plan (McNichol, 1989).

Colostomy Care. Colostomies are placed in infants because of an anorectal malformation (e.g., imperforate anus, rectal atresis) or Hirschsprung's disease (an absence of ganglia cells in an intestinal segment resulting in a lack of peristalsis). Older children may require colostomies for inflammatory bowel disease (ulcerative colitis or Crohn's disease). Ostomy care in infants under a year is usually done without an appliance, whereas older children will usually have an appliance. The use of a gauze square dressing placed over the ostomy and secured with a diaper is usually adequate for infants and toddlers. However, pediatric appliances are available if there are concerns regarding skin breakdown around the ostomy. Some parents will choose to alternate methods depending upon convenience and cost. As with adult ostomy care, there are many skin care creams, ointments, and powders available. Some trial and error may be necessary to determine which products are most effective for each individual child.

Before hospital discharge, the family must demonstrate total responsibility for ostomy care over a 24-hour period. The home care nurse should be aware of all teaching that was done in the hospital, the family's demonstrated abilities, and all supplies needed. Home care services for the child with an ostomy include

1. Home care nursing visits to assess knowledge level and teach ostomy care, various ostomy care techniques, ostomy irrigations, if ordered, skin care, symptoms of dehydration, expectations of volume and consistency of ostomy drainage, and growth and development
2. A consult with an enterostomal therapist may be needed to develop a final, comprehensive care plan with long-term issues considered

Pediatric Home Intravenous Therapy. Home IV therapy for children is a more recent development in high-tech pediatric home care, but it is often a viable and safe alternative to hospitalization. Intravenous therapy may be peripheral or central and serve the purpose of providing hydration, administration of antibiotics, pain medications, or chemotherapy, and IV therapy often is used for total parenteral nutrition. The success of home IV therapy for children is strongly dependent on client and family suitability. Not all clients who could be managed at home are able to meet eligibility criteria.

A critical aspect of pediatric home IV therapy is the predischarge planning and screening for eligibility to participate in the program. Screening criteria should include

1. Ability of client and family to demonstrate adequate skills
2. Minimal risk for abusing IV site or supplies
3. Backup plan for restarting peripheral IV
4. Family's life-style and environment suitability to supporting home IV
5. Clinical stability of child
6. Parents' signing of informed consent form to indicate understanding of their responsibilities for home IV

Prior to discharge the family must demonstrate complete responsibility for care of the IV over a 24-hour period. The home care nurse should be aware of all teaching done, the family's demonstrated abilities, and all equipment and supplies needed. Home care services for the child with an IV include

1. Home care nursing visits to teach and assess patency of IV site, IV complications, and the child's clinical response to the IV therapy
2. Home visits from equipment vendor to teach operation and maintenance of IV pumps (see generic care plan, Appendix 11)

Home Phototherapy. Home phototherapy is a proven safe and effective method for treating full-term newborns with physiological jaundice. The benefits of phototherapy are cost savings by reducing lengthy hospitalizations and an uninterrupted parent–infant attachment process. Families who receive careful screening and training have done well with home phototherapy programs (Wilkerson, 1989).

Before hospital discharge, families must demonstrate knowledge of necessary observations and procedures to follow while the infant is under the lights. Written instructions on infant care and equipment use are essential. To ensure that parents understand the care requirements, a signed teaching or consent form is used. Home care services for the child under home phototherapy include

1. Daily home care nursing visits to assess the status of the newborn and reinforce teaching with the family and to assess their continued ability to carry out home phototherapy safely
2. Home visits by the equipment vendor to teach operation and maintenance of lights
3. Home blood specimens drawn for laboratory testing (see generic care plan, Appendix 11)

Terminally Ill Children. The high-tech home care needs for terminally ill children can include many of the aspects of care discussed previously. The general considerations and overall services needed will be discussed in this section.

Home care for the terminally ill child has many advantages. Children are more tolerant of pain, discomfort, and fatigue when they are in familiar surroundings. Family members feel less loss of control when they are allowed to participate in the child's care and may cope more realistically with the impending death while experiencing the gradual decline of the child.

A terminally ill child can be kept at home if there is a parent or other caregiver willing to take responsibility for the child's care. Discharge planning should take into consideration the family's needs, resources, and ability to cope with the stress of home care. Home care services for the terminally ill child include

1. Home care nursing visits to assess and teach the family about pain management, nutrition, sleep and rest, elimination, skin care, and preparation for death
2. Social work visits to assist the family in coping with emotional, psychosocial, and financial concerns
3. Medical equipment and supply vendor to teach operation of equipment and service as necessary

General Considerations

Although each type of pediatric home care has its own unique aspects, there are several general considerations.

1. There are no specific visit frequencies for children. Visit frequency is individualized based on the teaching needs of the family and the acuity level of the child.
2. All home nursing services and equipment vendors must provide 24-hour availability.
3. Nurses must refer to other professionals, such as physical and speech therapists, social workers, nutritionists, and home health aides.
4. Nurses must keep open lines of communication with physicians and other personnel involved.
5. Respite care always must be available to family caregivers.

Family and caregiver burnout is always a possibility in pediatric home care. The home care nurse is in the best position to evaluate continually the appropriateness and safety of the home care plan. Families may forget that there are options to home care. It may be the nurse who suggests that home care may not be the optimal plan. Alternatives available can include long-term care in a skilled nursing facility or foster care, depending on community resources.

Community Resources

Sources of funding for pediatric home care can include the following

1. Private insurance and HMOs
2. Medicaid
3. Supplemental Security Income (SSI)
4. Women, Infants and Children Program (WIC)
5. Food stamps
6. State crippled children's services
7. State and local social service agencies
8. Community or disease specific organizations
9. Religious organizations
10. State and local public health and education programs
11. Private contributions

Sources of support and informational resources can be obtained from local chapters of many national organizations. Appendix 12 is a brief list of these organizations.

HOSPICE HOME CARE

The History of Hospice

The hospice concept was originated in medieval Europe, where places of refuge were provided for travelers as they journeyed to the many sites of pilgrimage, often with great hardship. As early as the nineteenth century, hospices in England provided palliative care to terminally ill patients in hospitals and then provided care in the client's home. Historically, dying has been viewed as a natural process in which family and friends provided all of the care that was needed. As the health care system became more complex and impersonal, the common place for death shifted from the home to the hospital. The experience of dying in a hospital has changed the nature of dying for both the client and the family. The need to humanize the health care system has made room for the development of the hospice concept.

In the United States, the impetus for the development of hospice care came in 1974 in New Haven, Connecticut, where a hospice was established starting with a home care program and then subsequently adding an inpatient facility. A group of professionals (doctors, nurses, social workers, clergy, etc.) and lay volunteers modeled this first American hospice after St. Christopher's Hospice in England. As the Connecticut hospice grew in the number of clients served and the types of care provided, there was the institution of paid professional care within the organization. Today, Connecticut Hospice is the first free-standing hospice in the United States, providing a model for terminal care that many organizations have followed.

The Hospice Philosophy

Today hospice refers to "a concept of care that is practiced anywhere by anyone when support is offered to people who are dying whether or not it is formally recognized as hospice care" (Sheehan, 1988). Most students of the hospice concept agree that it is a philosophy of care rather than a place of care. This means that hospice nursing can be provided in the home, a hospice inpatient facility, an acute care hospital, or an extended care facility. Although people prefer to stay at home with home care as the focus, the place of care is much less important than the type of care that is provided.

Hospice care couples the most up-to-date principles of pain control and symptom management with the centuries' old principles of compassionate, individualized care and concern for the dignity of the dying client. It is much more than the coordination of care from a variety of caregivers. The practice of hospice care revolves around careful attention to the physiological, psychosocial, and spiritual needs of the client and his or her significant others. The care usually begins sometime in the last 6 months of the client's life and extends through the bereavement period with the family.

The hospice nurse must possess a firm foundation in the home care principles and skills included in this book. Furthermore, the nurse working with hospice clients must function as a member of an interdisciplinary team, possess the ability to address the emotional needs of the hospice client and family, and have a broad knowledge of community resources (Stanhope & Lancaster, 1988).

Basic Tenets of the Hospice Philosophy. There are specific, recognizable elements that are part of all hospice programs and go beyond just medical care for the terminally ill. The basic tenets of the hospice philosophy are described by Lack (1979).

1. A comprehensive approach to care. Attention to the physiological, psychological, sociological, and spiritual needs of the client and family constellation is the focus of all care given to hospice clients. This also implies continuity of care, whether the client is at home or in an inpatient setting.

   A holistic approach to the client and the family are integral components of the hospice philosophy. The client and family benefit from the availability of skilled professionals trained to meet their physical, psychological, sociological, and spiritual needs.

2. Concentration on the client and family as the unit of service. Consistent with the philosophy of home care nursing, hospice care recognizes the family as the unit of care. As such, care is provided with the recognition that the family and the client must be the recipients of care. If the family is unable to cope emotionally with some aspect of the client situation, interventions should be provided to the family as well as the client. Recognition of the family's role in the provision of care is also a component of this principle. Hospice interventions may be focused on assisting the family in the development of the necessary skills to care for a dying relative.

3. An interdisciplinary team approach to care. The interdisciplinary team includes physicians, nurses, social workers, home health aides, spe-

cialized therapists, pastoral counselors, and clergy. Recognizing that one health professional cannot have all the answers, the collaboration of many health professionals is essential in meeting the complex needs of the dying client and his or her family. Working together as a team, services that most completely meet the needs of the client and family are provided.

Clients may not want or need the services of all members of the hospice team. All services are available to the client and family at any point in the client's illness, but the use of all services is not a requirement of hospice care.

The hospice home care nurse plays a major role as a member of the interdisciplinary team. Most commonly, the hospice nurse makes the initial home visit and identifies the client and family needs. As other disciplines become involved in the situation, the hospice nurse retains responsibility for the planning, implementation, evaluation, and coordination of the nursing care.

4. Utilization of direct service volunteers as part of the interdisciplinary team. The use of volunteers as part of the hospice interdisciplinary team originated in the early days of the hospice movement in the United States. Since hospice care was developed through the efforts of a volunteer workforce, the tradition of using volunteers continues to have a strong influence and is a requirement of the federal regulations concerning hospice. Volunteers provide a variety of services, including respite care, meal preparation, and friendly visiting.

5. Concentration of care on the improvement of the quality of life, not the extension of life. Pain and symptom control, elements of palliative care, are very important aspects of the hospice philosophy and are probably the elements with which clients are most familiar. Unlike health care that focuses on curing diseases, palliative care is described as care that focuses on the relief from symptoms and discomfort. For example, if an abdominal tumor is causing severe pain as a result of compression of organs, palliative care could involve relief of that pain through the use of analgesics rather than removal of the tumor through surgical intervention.

   Palliative care is fundamentally different from the chronic care model to which many home care nurses are accustomed. In the palliative care model, nothing is done "to the client" beyond those measures that relate to symptom control. The client and family have full authority in determining the care that will be provided. For example, monitoring the diet of a diabetic in his final weeks of life may not be done at all by the hospice nurse.

Vital signs may not be taken on a terminally ill cardiac client. This difference in approach may be difficult for nurses in agencies that serve both hospice clients and traditional home care clients. Recognition of the differences in nursing approaches will be helpful in meeting the needs of all clients and families.

Symptom control is achieved through noninvasive assessment of the client's problems followed by interventions that involve an individually titrated medication administration to control pain and retain alertness (Blues & Zerwekh, 1984.)

6. Service availability on an 24-hour, 7 day per week basis. The type of care required by dying clients and their families is not restricted to an 8-hour period during the day. Many clients feel most frightened and alone at night when the visitors have left and the environment is quiet. For hospice clients and their families, around the clock availability of professionals and services is essential to help the family feel that they can cope with situations that arise. This constant availability often makes the difference between keeping clients at home or admitting them to the hospital (Jarvis, 1985).

7. Bereavement follow-up. Bereavement care is available to the family, usually for 1 year following the death of the client or until services are no longer needed or wanted. Services include helping the family adjust to the emotional, social, spiritual, and economic changes that come as a result of the death of a loved one. Bereavement services can be provided in the form of individual home visits with the family, self-help groups, or therapeutic groups led by a professional. Families may determine which strategy they feel would be most comforting and beneficial.

The Medicare Hospice Benefit

Like home care agencies, hospice providers must bill for the services provided to their clients so they can remain fiscally solvent. The regulations and restrictions that are part of the traditional Medicare program are not well suited to the terminally ill client. As such, legislation was enacted in 1983 that resulted in the development of a Medicare hospice benefit for terminally ill clients.

In order for a client to be admitted to a hospice program, regardless of the payment source, certain admission criteria must be considered. For home care services, the usual admission criteria include

1. A diagnosis of a terminal illness
2. A prognosis of 6 months or less

3. Informed consent to have hospice services on the part of the client
4. A referral by the client's physician

When a client elects to use the Medicare hospice benefit (inpatient or home care), he or she must waive the traditional Medicare benefit. In doing this, the client is eligible to receive several services and resources that were unavailable previously. The hospice benefit is available to the client for a period of 210 days only. Therefore, the criterion of a prognosis of 6 months or less is very important. If a client uses the 210 day hospice Medicare benefit prematurely, he or she will have access only to traditional Medicare when more extensive terminal care resources are really needed. A client must meet all Medicare criteria for home care, except be homebound, to be eligible for the hospice Medicare benefit. The hospice Medicare benefit covers

- Nursing, home health aide, and social work visits deemed necessary by the hospice care team
- Services, including pastoral care, dietary counseling, and other supportive programs
- Therapy services, such as physical therapy, deemed necessary by the hospice care team
- Prescription drugs related to the condition requiring hospice care are covered at the rate of 95% of cost
- Durable medical equipment needed for hospice home care is covered 100%

Types of Hospice Providers

There are many methods of providing hospice care to clients. Some agencies offer only services for the client in their home, while other providers couple home care with inpatient hospital services. Recognizing that the hospice concept is a philosophy of care rather than a place where care is given, it seems appropriate that hospice care can be given in a variety of settings. The following are the commonly seen types of hospice care providers.

1. A home care agency, certified as a hospice provider, delivers care to the terminally ill client in the home. Care is provided to the hospice clients using the interdisciplinary team approach.
2. An independent agency that serves hospice clients exclusively. These agencies are licensed as home care agencies and are certified as hospice providers. Some of these independent agencies have inpatient facilities, while others contract with local hospitals for the care of acutely ill clients.
3. An acute care hospital may have either hospice units or specially designated hospice beds. When

the client is discharged from the hospital, home care is provided by one of the other types of hospice home care providers.

In summary, hospice care is a philosophy that is a humane alternative for terminally ill clients. Using an interdisciplinary team approach, terminal care that focuses on palliative care, specific symptom control, emotional support, and pain management is provided to the clients and their families. Recognizing the complex needs of the dying client and his or her family, care is focused on meeting their physiological, psychological, social, and spiritual needs. Clients receiving hospice care can waive their traditional Medicare benefit for a more comprehensive hospice Medicare benefit that is designed to meet their health care needs.

TEST YOURSELF

1. What issues must be considered before sending a high-tech client home from the hospital? What are the similarities and differences to consider when the client is a child?

2. When visiting a client who is receiving enteral feedings, you assess that the client has nausea and vomiting. What interventions, including client teaching, would you incorporate into your care plan?

3. Identify one high-tech pediatric illness you see in your agency (or have read about in this or another book). Identify the services needed to keep this pediatric client at home.

4. Describe in your own words how hospice care differs from traditional care of a terminally ill client.

5. What steps would you take to refer a client to a hospice provider in your community?

6. Describe the differences between the traditional Medicare benefit and the Medicare hospice benefit.

REFERENCES

Chapter 1

American Colleges of Physicians Health and Public Policy Committee (1986). Home health care position paper. *Annals of Internal Medicine, 105,* 454–460.

Clemen-Stone, S., Eigsti, D.G. & McGuire, S.L. (1987). *Comprehensive Family and Community Health Nursing* (2nd ed.) New York: McGraw-Hill.

Friedman, J. (1986). *Home Health Care: A Complete Guide for Patients and Their Families.* New York: W.W. Norton.

Harris, M.D. (1988). *Home Health Administration.* Owings Mills, MD: National Health Publishing.

Humphrey, C.J. (1988). The home as a setting for care—clarifying the boundaries of practice. *Nursing Clinics of North America, 223,* 305–314.

National Association for Home Care (1987). *How To Choose a Home Care Agency.* Washington DC.

Nassif, J.F. (1985) *The Home Health Care Solution.* Mount Vernon, NY: Consumers Union.

Chapter 2

Berg, R. (Ed.) (1988) *The APIC Curriculum for Infection Control Practice.* Dubuque Iowa: Kendall/Hunt Publishing. Copyrighted information, used with permission.

Gordon, M. (1976). Nursing diagnosis and diagnostic process. *American Journal of Nursing, 76,* 1298–1300.

Home care nursing services (1988). *Caring, 7,* 8–9.

Humphrey, C. (1986) *Home Care Nursing Handbook.* E. Norwalk, Ct: Appleton-Century-Crofts.

Iyer, P., Taptich, B. & Bernocchi-Losey, D. (1986). *Nursing Process and Nursing Diagnosis.* Philadelphia: W.B. Saunders.

McFarland, G. & McFarlane, E. (1989). *Nursing Diagnosis and Intervention.* St. Louis, Mo: C.V. Mosby.

Mundinger, M., Jauron, G. (1975). Developing a nursing diagnosis. *Nursing Outlook, 33,* 94–98.

Mundinger, M.O. (1983). *Home Care Controversy: Too Little, Too Late, Too Costly.* Rockville, MD: Aspen.

Scott, B., Trusler, M., & Simmons, B. (1988). Infection Control Guidelines for Home Health. Washington, DC: National Association for Home Care Working Paper.

Health-care settings. *Morbidity and Mortality Weekly Report,* (1988). 37, 377–382.

Chapter 3

American Nurses' Association (1985). *Standards for Home Care Nursing.* Kansas City, Mo.

Barlow, A. (1989) Comprehensive quality assurance. *Caring, 7,* 17–19.

Collins v Westlake, 57 Ill 2d 388, 312 N.E. 614.

Crawford v. Earl Long Memorial Hospital, et al., La App 1 Cir (1983), 431 So.2d. 70 (1983).

Frankenburg, W.K., & Dodds, J.B. (1978). *Denver Developmental Screening Test* (DDST). University of Colorado Medical Center.

Helberg, J. (1983). Documentation in child abuse. *American Journal of Nursing, 83,* 223–239.

Humphrey, C. (1986). *Home Care Nursing Handbook.* E. Norwalk, Ct: Appleton-Century-Crofts.

Medicare Home Health Agency Manual Pub 11. (April, 1989). Washington, DC: Home Care Financing Administrations.

Phaneuf, M. (1976). Documentation of the side effects of medication. *Home Health Care Nurse, 5,* 36–38.

Pisel v. Stamford Hospital, 180 Conn. 314, 430 A. 2d (1980).

Plastaras, S. (1987). Documentation of the side effects of medication. *Home Health Care Nurse, 5,* 36–38.

Scappatura v. Baptist Hospital, 120 Ariz. 204, 584 P. 2d1195 (1978).

Utter v. United Hospital Center, 236 S.E. 2d 213 (W. Va., 1977).

Wagner v. Kaiser Foundation Hospitals, 185 Or. 81, 589 p. 2d 1106 (1979).

Wisnom, B (1989). Quality assurance: Is your practice effective? In Dittmar, S. *Rehabilitation Nursing,* St. Louis, Mo: C.V. Mosby

Chapter 4

Aleman, A. (1982). Nursing care of the multiproblem poor family *Home Health Care Nurse, 1,* 34–38.

Benefield, L. (1988). *Home Health Care Management.* Englewood Cliffs, NJ: Prentice Hall.

Bloom, B. (1969). *Taxonomy of Educational Objectives.* New York: David McKay.

Cohn, V. (1988, June 21, 22). The impact on you of managed care *The Washington Post.*

Desimone, B. (1988, July). The case for case management. *Continuing Care,* 22–23.

Doak, C., Doak. L., & Root, J. (1985). *Teaching Patients With Low Literacy Skills.* Philadelphia: J.B. Lippincott.

Humphrey, C. (1986). *Home Care Nursing Handbook.* E. Norwalk, Ct: Appleton-Century-Crofts.

Hussey, L., & Gilliland, K. (1989). Compliance, low literacy and locus of control. *Nursing Clinics of North America 25,* 605–611.

Jackson, J., & Johnson, E. (1988). *Patient Education in Home Care.* Rockville, MD: Aspen.

Knollmueller, R. (1989). Case management: What's in a name? *Nursing Management, 20,* 38–40.

Knowles, M. (1980). *The Modern Practice of Adult Education.* Chicago, Il: Follett.

Leff, E. (1986). Ethics and patient teaching. *The American Journal of Maternal—Child Nursing. 11,* 375–378.

Marquis, B., & Huston, C. (1987). *Management Decision Making for Nurses.* Philadelphia, PA: J.B. Lippincott.

Medicare Home Health Agency Manual Pub. 11. (April 1989). Washington, DC: Home Care Financing Administration.

Omdahl, D. (1987). Preventing home care denials. *American Journal of Nursing, 8,* 1031–1033.

Patterson, O. (ed) (1962). *Special Tools for Communication.* Chicago, IL: Industrial Audio-Visual Association.

Sloan, M., & Schommer, B. (1982). The process of contracting in community health nursing. In Spradley, B. (Ed.) *Readings In Community Health Nursing* Boston, Ma: Little, Brown. 241–248.

Spradley, B.W. (1985). *Community Health Nursing.* Boston, Ma: Little, Brown.

Stanhope, M, & Lancaster, J. (1988). *Community Health Nursing.* St. Louis, Mo: C.V. Mosby.

Chapter 5

Case, T. (1986). *Work Stresses of Community Health Nurses.* Unpublished master's thesis, University of Oklahoma City, OK.

Cestari, L.R. (1989). *A Comparison of Stress among Hospital and Community Health Nurses.* Unpublished master's thesis, Southern Connecticut State University, New Haven, Ct.

Hache-Faulkner, N. (1983). *A Comparison of Stress and its Major Sources in Public Health and Hospital Nursing as Perceived by Staff Nurses.* Unpublished master's research, Dalhousie University, Halifax, Nova Scotia, Canada.

Myers, M.B. (1988). Home care nursing: A view from the field. *Public Health Nursing, 5,* 65–67.

Reemtsma, J.T. (Producer) (1981). *Nurse, Where Are You?* [Film]. New York: CBS News.

Chapter 6

American Nurses' Association. (1985). *Code for Nurses With Interpretive Statements.* Kansas City, MO.

American Nurses' Association (1987). *Liability and You—What Registered Nurses Need to Know.* Kansas City, MO.

American Nurses' Association (1986). *Standards for Home Care Nursing.* Kansas City, MO.

American Nurses' Association (1986). *Standards of Community Health Nursing Practice.* Kansas City, MO.

American Nurses' Association. (1986). *Standards of Nursing Practice.* Kansas City, MO.

Bass v. Barksdale et al., 671 S.W. 2d 476 (Tenn App. 1984).

Connaway, N. (1985). Documenting patient care in the home-legal issues for the home health nurse (pt. ii). *Home Health Care Nurse.* 3, 44–46.

Connaway, N. (1986). Incident reports in home health agencies. *Home Health Care Nurse*, 4, 9–10.

Cushing, M. (1982). The legal side: A matter of judgment. *American Journal of Nursing* 990–992.

Czubinsky v. Doctor's Hospital, 139 Cal. App. 3d 361, 188 Cal 685 (1983).

Guigino v. Harvard Community Health Plan et al., 403 N.E. 2d 1166 (Mass., 1980).

Josberger, M.C. & Ries, D.T. (1985). Nurse experts—selecting and preparing them for litigation. *Trial, 21*, 68–71.

Killion, S. (1985). Patients' rights to their medical records. *Health Span, 2*, 28–33.

Northrop, C., & Kelly, M. (1987). *Legal Issues in Nursing.* St. Louis, MO: C.V. Mosby.

Pisel v. Stanford Hospital, 180 Conn. 314, 430 A. 2d (1980).

Rivers v. Katz, 504 N.Y.S 2d 74, 495 N.E. 2d 337 (1986).

Sandroff, R. (1983). Why you really ought to have your own malpractice policy. *RN, 46*, 29–33.

Utter v. United Hospital Center, 236 S.E. 2d 213 (W. Va., 1977).

Chapter 7

Ahmann, E. (1986). *Home Care For the High-Risk Infant.* Rockville, MD: Aspen.

Blues, A., & Zerwekh, J. (1984). *Hospice and Palliative Nursing Care.* New York: Grune & Stratton.

Cabin, B. (1985). Cost effectiveness of pediatric home care. *Caring, 4*, 45–53.

Feinburg, E. (1985). Family stress in pediatric home care. *Caring, 5*, 38–41.

Goldberg, A., Faure, E., Vaughn, C., Sharski, R., & Seleny, F. (May, 1984). Home care for life supported persons: An approach to program development, *Journal of Pediatrics, 104*(5), 785–795.

Grammatica, G. (1989). Developing a quality home care program for children. *Pediatric Nursing, 15*, 33–35.

Hartsell, M., & Ward, J. (1985). Selecting equipment vendors for children on home care. MCN: *The American Journal of Maternal—Child Nursing, 10*, 26–28.

Heiser, C. (1987). Home phototherapy. *Pediatric Nursing, 13*, 425–427.

Home care for the perinatal, neonatal, and pediatric client. (1987, Spring). *Health Source, XI.*

Jarvis, L. (1985). *Community Health Nursing: Keeping the Public Healthy* (2nd ed.). Philadelphia, Pa: F.A. Davis.

Kennedy, A.H., Johnson, W., & Sturdevant, E. (1982). An educational program for families of children with tracheostomies. MCN: *The American Journal of Maternal—Child Nursing, 7*, 42–49.

Klijanowicz, A. (1985). Home apnea monitoring. *NAACOG Update Series.* Vol. 3, Lesson 15, pp 2–7.

Kun, S., & Brennan, K. (1985). Pediatric discharge planning: Challenges and rewards. *Caring, 4*, 37.

Lack, S.A. (1979). Hospice: A concept of care in the final stage of life. *Connecticut Medicine, 3*, 365–369.

Macmarik, R., & Thompson, J. (1986). Respiratory care of the ventilator-assisted infant in the home. *Respiratory Care, 31*, 605.

McNichol, J. (1989). When eating doesn't come naturally. *MCN: The American Journal of Maternal—Child Nursing, 1*(14), 23–26.

Sheehan, C. (1988). Hospice licensure: A philosophical and conceptual framework. *Caring, 7*, 8–11.

Stanhope, M., & Lancaster, J. (1988). *Community Health Nursing* (2nd ed.). St Louis, MO: C.V. Mosby.

Wilkerson, M.N. (1989) Treating Hyperbilirubinemia. *MCN: The American Journal of Maternal—Child Nursing*, (14)1, 32–36.

Additional Resources

A.S.P.E.N., Board of directors. (1987). Guidelines for use of home total parenteral nutrition. *Journal of Parenteral and Enteral Nutrition, 11*, 342–344.

Baird, S., Hartgans, R., & Smith, D. (1987). *The Role of the Oncology Nurse* in *the Office Setting.* Adria Laboratories.

Bazigin, E. (April, 1987). Stability of antineoplastics. *The Home Health Care Professional*, Vol. iv, No. 1, pl.

Bedrosian, C.A. (1989). *Home Health Nursing: Nursing Diagnoses and Care Plans.* E. Norwalk, Ct: Appleton & Lange.

Blackburn, G.L., & Baptista, R.J. (1984). Home TPN: State of the art. *American Journal of Intravenous & Clinical Nutrition*, 20–32.

Bulau, J. (1989). *Quality Assurance Policies and Procedures for Home Health Care.* Rockville, MD: Aspen.

Carlson, R.V., & Brandimir, I. (1983). Continuous infusion or bolus injection in cancer chemotherapy. *Annals of Internal Medicine, 99*, 823–833.

Devaney, S., & Diehm, C. (1989, September). Orientation and training: Their role in staff retention. *Caring.* 24–27.

Eisenberg, J.M., & Kitz, D.S. (1986). Savings from outpatient antibiotic therapy for osteomyelitis. *JAMA, 255*, 1584–1589.

Ethridge, D. (1989). Professional nursing case management improves quality, access and costs. *Nursing Management, 20*, 30–35.

Gould, E.J., & Nargo, J. (1987). *Home Health Nursing Care Plans.* Rockville, MD: Aspen.

Hache-Faulkner, N., & MacKay, R.C. (1985). Stress in the workplace: Public health and hospital nurses. *Canadian Nurse. 81.* 40–42.

Hays, J. (1989). Voices in the record. *Image, 21*, 200–204.

Hinshaw, A.S., Smeltzer, C., & Atwood, J.R. (1987). Innovative retention strategies for nursing staff. *JONA, 17*, 6.

Huffman, K.C. (1989). Psychosocial concerns of home nutrition therapy consumers. *Nutrition in Clinical Practice, 4*, 51–56.

Jacob, S. (1985). The impact of documentation in home health care. *Home Health Care Nurse, 3*, 16–19.

Jaffe, M.S., & Skidmore-Roth, L. (1988). *Home Health Nursing Care Plans.* St. Louis, MO: C.V. Mosby.

Johnson, E., & Jackson, J. (1989). Teaching the home care client. *Nursing Clinics of North America, 24*, 687–693.

Keating, S.B., & Kelman, G.B. (1988). *Home Health Care Nursing: Concepts and Practice.* Philadelphia, Pa: J.B. Lippincott.

Kerfoot, K. (1988). Retention: What's it all about? *Nursing Economics, 6*, 42–43.

Kirk, R., & Kranz, D. (1988). *Home Care Management.* Rockville, MD: Aspen.

Knollmueller, R.N. (1979). What happened to the PHN supervisor? *Nursing Outlook, 27*, 666.

Knollmueller, R.N. (1986). *The Community Health Nursing Supervisor. A Handbook for Community/Home Care Managers.* New York, NY: National League for Nursing, 21–1999.

Knollmueller, R.N. (1987). Educational needs of home health agency supervisors. Quality and Home Health Care: Redefining the tradition. A special publication of the *Quality Review Bulletin*, Chicago, IL: Joint Commission on Accreditation of Healthcare Organizations. pp. 83–86.

Knollmueller, R.N. (1988). Reshaping supervisory Practice in Home Care. *Nursing Clinics of North America*, 353–362. Vol 23, No 2.

Malloy, C., & Hartshorn, J. (1989). *Acute Care Nursing in the Home: A Holistic Approach.* Philadelphia, Pa: J.B. Lippincott.

Marrelli, T.M. (1988). *Handbook of Home Health Standards & Documentation Guidelines for Reimbursement.* St. Louis, MD, C.V. Mosby.

Martinson, I., & Widmer, A. (1989). *Home Health Care Nursing.* Philadelphia, Pa: W.B. Saunders.

Meisenheimer, C. (1988). *Client Teaching Guides for Home Health Care.* Rockville, MD: Aspen.

Mooney, V., Diver, B., Schnackel, A. (1988). Developing a cost-effective clinical preceptorship program. *Journal of Nursing Administration, 18*(1), 31–36.

Morrissey-Ross, M. (1988). Documentation, If you haven't written it, you haven't done it. *Nursing Clinics of North America, 23,* 363–372.

O'Hare, P., & Terry, M. (eds.) (1987). *Discharge Planning for Continuity of Care,* Rockville, MD: Aspen.

Omdahl, D. (1988). Home care charting do's and don'ts. *American Journal of Nursing, 88,* 203–204.

Parsons, P. (1986). Building better treatment plans. *Journal of Psychosocial Nursing, 24,* 9–14.

Piemme, J., Tack, B., Kramer, W., Evans, J. (1986). Developing the nurse preceptor. *The Journal of Continuing Education in Nursing, 17,* No6, 186–189.

Prato, S.A. (1987). Effective nursing orientation can thwart dissatisfaction. *Health Progress, 67,* 49–52.

Reardon, J., McSweeney, M., & O'Neill, E. (1987). Continuous infusion of 5-fluoracil with concomitant in esophageal carcinoma. *The Home Health Care Professional,* IVF(1).

Reardon, J. (1987). Providing total care for the cancer patient and family: A challenge for the home care team. *The Home Care Professional,* IV(1).

Sandrick, K. (1986). Home care: Cutting health care's safety net. *Hospitals, 5,* 48–52.

Shamansky, S.L. (1988). Home health care. *Nursing Clinics of North America, 23.*

Treloar, D. (1986). Cephalosporins—third generation. *RN 1,* 28–32.

Wagner, D. (1988). *Managing for quality in home health care.* Rockville, MD: Aspen.

Watterworth, B., & Podrasky, D. (1989). Meeting the learning needs of the person discharged home with an open wound. *Journal of Enterostomal Therapy, 16,* 12–15.

Wilhelm, L. (1985). Helping your patient 'settle in' with TPN. *Nursing 85,* 60–64.

Zastocki, D., & Rovinski, C. (1989). *Home care, patient and family instructions.* Philadelphia: W.B. Saunders.

Windshield Survey

A tour of your community in your car is one way to get an overview of the characteristics, housing, resources, residents, and industry. By looking carefully at these community characteristics, you can begin to get a flavor for the types of clients you will be serving. For example, if you notice posters and billboards in Spanish as you drive around the community, you can assume that there is a significant Spanish-speaking population in your service area. This observation will need to be validated through collection of additional data.

The social and economic levels of the community can be identified in a windshield survey. As you observe the community, you will notice not only the type of housing but the quality and its condition. Housing in poor condition may be indicative of a depressed economic environment or the presence of debilitated elderly persons who are unable to maintain a house. On your windshield survey you may also identify significant barriers to healthy living. For example, you may observe many homes with the windows open without screens in place. In addition to the problem of flies and other insects in the house windows without screens pose a significant safety hazard for young children.

A windshield survey will only give the home care nurse a broad view of the community To develop an in-depth understanding of the characteristics and the dynamics of the community, a detailed community assessment is indicated.

In a 1-hour tour of your service area observe the following community characteristics:

1. Housing
2. Cultural and ethnic factors
3. Industry and business
4. Population
5. Resources (e.g., churches, self-help groups)

NANDA Approved Nursing Diagnostic Categories

(as published in the Summer 1988 NANDA Nursing Diagnosis Newsletter)

This list represents the NANDA approved nursing diagnostic categories for clinical use and testing (1988). Changes have been made in 15 labels for consistency.

PATTERN 1: EXCHANGING

1.1.2.1	Altered Nutrition: More than body requirements
1.1.2.2	Altered Nutrition: Less than body requirements
1.1.2.3	Altered Nutrition: Potential for more than body requirements
1.2.1.1	Potential for Infection
1.2.2.1	Potential Altered Body Temperature
**1.2.2.2	Hypothermia
1.2.2.3	Hyperthermia
1.2.2.4	Ineffective Thermoregulation
*1.2.3.1	Dysreflexia
#1.3.1.1	Constipation
*1.3.1.1.1	Perceived Constipation
*1.3.1.1.2	Colonic Constipation
#1.3.1.2	Diarrhea
#1.3.1.3	Bowel Incontinence
1.3.2	Altered Urinary Elimination
1.3.2.1.1	Stress Incontinence
1.3.2.1.2	Reflex Incontinence
1.3.2.1.3	Urge Incontinence
1.3.2.1.4	Functional Incontinence
1.3.2.1.5	Total Incontinence
1.3.2.2	Urinary Retention
#1.4.1.1	Altered (Specify Type) Tissue Perfusion (Renal, cerebral, cardiopulmonary, gastrointestinal, peripheral)
1.4.1.2.1	Fluid Volume Excess
1.4.1.2.2.1	Fluid Volume Deficit
1.4.1.2.2.2	Potential Fluid Volume Deficit
#1.4.2.1	Decreased Cardiac Output
1.5.1.1	Impaired Gas Exchange
1.5.1.2	Ineffective Airway Clearance
1.5.1.3	Ineffective Breathing Pattern
1.6.1	Potential for Injury
1.6.1.1	Potential for Suffocation
1.6.1.2	Potential for Poisoning
1.6.1.3	Potential for Trauma
*1.6.1.4	Potential for Aspiration
*1.6.1.5	Potential for Disuse Syndrome
1.6.2.1	Impaired Tissue Integrity
#1.6.2.1.1	Altered Oral Mucous Membrane
1.6.2.1.2.1	Impaired Skin Integrity
1.6.2.1.2.2	Potential Impaired Skin Integrity

PATTERN 2: COMMUNICATING

2.1.1.1	Impaired Verbal Communication

PATTERN 3: RELATING

3.1.1	Impaired Social Interaction
3.1.2	Social Isolation
#3.2.1	Altered Role Performance
3.2.1.1.1	Altered Parenting
3.2.1.1.2	Potential Altered Parenting
3.2.1.2.1	Sexual Dysfunction
3.2.2	Altered Family Processes
*3.2.3.1	Parental Role Conflict
3.3	Altered Sexuality Patterns

PATTERN 4: VALUING

4.1.1	Spiritual Distress (distress of the human spirit)

PATTERN 5: CHOOSING

5.1.1.1	Ineffective Individual Coping
5.1.1.1.1	Impaired Adjustment
*5.1.1.1.2	Defensive Coping
*5.1.1.1.3	Ineffective Denial
5.1.2.1.1	Ineffective Family Coping: Disabling
5.1.2.1.2	Ineffective Family Coping: Compromised
5.1.2.2	Family Coping: Potential for Growth
5.2.1.1	Noncompliance (Specify)
*5.3.1.1	Decisional Conflict (Specify)
*5.4	Health Seeking Behaviors (Specify)

PATTERN 6: MOVING

6.1.1.1	Impaired Physical Mobility
6.1.1.2	Activity Intolerance

*6.1.1.2.1	Fatigue
6.1.1.3	Potential Activity Intolerance
6.2.1	Sleep Pattern Disturbance
6.3.1.1	Diversional Activity Deficit
6.4.1.1	Impaired Home Maintenance Management
6.4.2	Altered Health Maintenance
#6.5.1	Feeding Self Care Deficit
6.5.1.1	Impaired Swallowing
*6.5.1.2	Ineffective Breastfeeding
#6.5.2	Bathing/Hygiene Self Care Deficit
#6.5.3	Dressing/Grooming Self Care Deficit
#6.5.4	Toileting Self Care Deficit
6.6	Altered Growth and Development

PATTERN 7: PERCEIVING

#7.1.1	Body Image Disturbance
#**7.1.2	Self Esteem Disturbance
*7.1.2.1	Chronic Low Self Esteem
*7.1.2.2	Situational Low Self Esteem
#7.1.3	Personal Identity Disturbance
7.2	Sensory/Perceptual Alterations (Specify) (Visual, auditory, kinesthetic, gustatory, tactile, olfactory)

7.2.1.1	Unilateral Neglect
7.3.1	Hopelessness
7.3.2	Powerlessness

PATTERN 8: KNOWING

8.1.1	Knowledge Deficit (Specify)
8.3	Altered Thought Processes

PATTERN 9: FEELING

#9.1.1	Pain
9.1.1.1	Chronic Pain
9.2.1.1	Dysfunctional Grieving
9.2.1.2	Anticipatory Grieving
9.2.2	Potential for Violence: Self-directed or directed at others
9.2.3	Post-Trauma Response
9.2.3.1	Rape-Trauma Syndrome
9.2.3.1.1	Rape-Trauma Syndrome: Compound Reaction
9.2.3.1.2	Rape-Trauma Syndrome: Silent Reaction
9.3.1	Anxiety
9.3.2	Fear

*New diagnostic categories approved 1988
**Revised diagnostic categories approved 1988
#Categories with modified label terminology.

Standardized Care Plan

CORONARY ARTERY DISEASE: ANGINA PECTORIS/MYOCARDIAL INFARCTION

Potential Complications

1. arrhythmias,
2. congestive heart failure,
3. thromboembolism,
4. Dressler's syndrome (post-MI syndrome),
5. cardiogenic shock,
6. ventricular aneurysm or rupture,
7. sudden death.

Types of Clients/Clinical Conditions Seen by Home Health Agencies

1. Persistent or recurrent chest pain; instruction and evaluation of client's response to newly ordered or changing medications; reporting significant changes in cardiac status to physician.
2. Recent MI: discharged home with inclusive teaching program regarding prescribed post-MI rehabilitation and treatment regimen.
3. Post-MI client with an unstable cardiovascular status, requiring changes in prescribed medications and treatment regimen: need for instruction and assessment of response to therapy changes.
4. Discharged home after hospitalization for post-MI complications.

Long-Term Goal

To meet the metabolic demands of the body and maintain optimal cardiac function through restoration of balance between oxygen demand and supply.

Short-Term Goals

The client with coronary artery disease: angina pectoris/myocardial infarction will be able to:

From Bedrosian, C.A. (1989). Home health nursing: Nursing diagnoses and care plans. E. Norwalk, CT: Appleton & Lange, with permission.

1. Verbalize nature of disease process, risk factors, S&S of new or recurring complications to report to home health nurse or physician.
2. Take pulse rate/describe alterations in rate or rhythm to report to physician.
3. Verbalize importance of well-balanced diet with prescribed dietary restrictions.
4. Demonstrate compliance with prescribed medication therapy/identify complications, toxicity.
5. Verbalize importance of taking pulse before taking digitalis, when to hold medication and call physician.
6. Verbalize/demonstrate compliance with prescribed anticoagulant therapy, safety precautions with use, adverse reactions to report to physician
7. Verbalize purpose of prescribed blood work.
8. Verbalize factors that precipitate angina/identify measures to relieve chest pain or require calling physician if pain persists.
9. Verbalize characteristics of MI and angina pectoris and actions to take with each/verbalize S&S to report to home health nurse or physician.
10. Demonstrate compliance with graded exercise program and activities/verbalize allowances and restrictions within the threshold of cardiac limitations, and of planned rest periods.
11. Demonstrate correct use of prescribed oxygen therapy/identify safety principles with use.
12. Verbalize understanding/identify measures to decrease dryness and breakdown of oral mucous membrane when on oxygen therapy.
13. Verbalize purpose/demonstrate correct use and application of antiembolic stocking.
14. Verbalize importance of not straining at stool and of prescribed measures to improve bowel functioning.
15. Verbalize importance of/wear Medic Alert bracelet.
16. Verbalize how to summon help in an emergency situation.
17. Exhibit decreased level of anxiety and apprehension with positive adaptation to cardiac condition.

Related Nursing Diagnosis

Activity Intolerance

related to:
Imbalance between oxygen supply and demand

as seen by:
Fatigue; weakness; abnormal heart and respiratory rate and BP in response to activity; exertional dyspnea; chest pain

Anxiety

related to:
1. Increase in anginal attacks with partial relief from nitrates and rest
2. Altered body image and life-style changes
3. Fear of recurrent "heart attack" and death
4. Knowledge deficit regarding prescribed home-care treatment regimen

as seen by:
Increased facial tension and apprehension; expressed fearfulness regarding heart condition and effect on life; increased questioning of managing at home post-MI

Bowel Elimination, Alteration in: Constipation

related to:
1. Prescribed activity restrictions
2. Inadequate dietary fiber and fluid intake

as seen by:
Straining at stool; frequency and amount less than usual pattern

Breathing Pattern, Ineffective

related to:
1. Chest pain
2. Decreased energy or fatigue

as seen by:
Exertional dyspnea; shortness of breath, altered depth of respiration; verbal report of fatigue

Cardiac Output, Alterations in: Decreased

related to:
Decreased myocardial contractility and altered conductivity secondary to myocardial damage

as seen by:
Weakness and fatigue, irregular heart rate; dizziness; restlessness; chest pain; changes in mental status

Comfort, Alteration in: Pain

related to:
Myocardial ischemia

as seen by:
c/o Restlessness; chest pain; apprehension; guarding behavior; diaphoresis; BP and pulse rate changes; increased or decreased respiratory rate

Gas Exchange, Impaired

related to:
Altered oxygen supply secondary to
1. Decreased cardiac output
2. Ineffective breathing patterns

as seen by:
Dyspnea; irritability; restlessness; cough; rales; pink, frothy sputum

Grieving

related to:
"Heart attack" and alteration in body image and life-style changes

as seen by:
Alterations in activity level; verbalization of distress over cardiac condition and effect on life; anger

Knowledge Deficit (Specify)

related to:
1. Disease process and related S&S
2. Prescribed plan of treatment for management of cardiac condition
3. Potential complications and S&S to report to home health nurse or physician

as seen by:
Verbalization of lack of information, inadequate understanding; inability to perform skills necessary to meet health-care needs at home

Injury, Potential for: Increased Risk of Falls and Injuries

related to:
1. Generalized weakness posthospitalization
2. Dizziness
3. Changes in mental status

as seen by:
Unsteady gait, weakness and fatigue; changes in alertness

Mobility, Impaired Physical

related to:
1. Activity intolerance
2. Chest pain
3. Prescribed activity restrictions

as seen by:
Weakness and fatigue; decreased endurance; reluctance to attempt movement; medically imposed restrictions

Oral Mucous Membrane, Alteration in

related to:
Dehydration of oral mucous membrane secondary to oxygen therapy

as seen by:
Oral pain or discomfort; thirst; coated tongue; halitosis

Self-Care Deficit: Feeding, Bathing/Hygiene, Dressing/Grooming, Toileting (Specify)

related to:
1. Activity intolerance
2. Impaired physical mobility
3. Prescribed activity restrictions

as seen by:
Reluctance to participate in daily activities and meet self-care needs, associated with weakness and fatigue; chest pain; exertional dyspnea

Nursing Actions/Treatments

1. Assess cardiovascular status/identify complications.
2. Assess vital signs/identify trends (e.g., hypo- or hypertension, pulse deficit)/instruct how to take and record pulse and about alterations in rate and rhythm to report to physician.
3. Instruct about nature of disease process (e.g., CAD, angina pectoris, MI), risk factors (e.g., obesity, smoking, stress, diet high in saturated fat and cholesterol, inactivity), importance of compliance with prescribed treatment regimen, S&S of complications to report to physician.
4. Assess and evaluate nutritional status/instruct about prescribed diet with restrictions (e.g., sodium, saturated fats and cholesterol, calories, caffeine)/obtain dietary consultation as needed.
5. Observe/instruct about taking medications as ordered, purpose and action, side effects, toxicity/ evaluate medication effectiveness.
6. Observe/instruct to take resting pulse for 1 minute before taking digitalis and to notify physician if pulse rate is below 60 or above 120 beats per minute or more irregular than usual before taking medication.

7. Assess/instruct about anticoagulant therapy, safety precautions to reduce risk of bleeding (e.g., avoid straining at stool; hard-bristled toothbrushes; aspirin or aspirin-containing products), adverse reactions to report to physician (e.g., bleeding, including bruises and petechial, hematuria, tarry stools)/educate regarding measures to control any bleeding (e.g., apply firm manual pressure for 10 minutes).
8. Monitor/instruct about purpose of prescribed blood work (e.g., coagulation times, digitalis levels, arterial blood gas analysis, cardiac enzyme levels to screen for evidence of progression of MI and need to rehospitalize).
9. Assess and evaluate clinical manifestations associated with angina pectoris, circumstances under which it occurs, factors that may precipitate it (e.g., specific activities; temperature extremes; emotional stress; nicotine)/instruct to modify activities, rest and take prescribed nitrates, call physician if pain persists.
10. Assess/instruct about patterns of chest pain (e.g., angina compared to MI), actions to take with each, S&S to report to home health nurse or physician.
11. Observe and evaluate level of physical tolerance to perform self-care activities and ADL (e.g., angina, exertional dyspnea, fatigue, excess anxiety)/ instruct about graded exercises and activities, allowances and restrictions within threshold of cardiac limitations/planned rest periods.
12. Observe/instruct about prescribed oxygen therapy: delivery method, flow rate, duration, care of equipment, safety principles with use (e.g., danger of smoking near oxygen system), care of equipment, obtain respiratory consultation as needed/evaluate effectiveness of oxygen therapy.
13. Assess and evaluate oral mucous membrane for dryness and breakdown when on oxygen therapy/instruct about good oral hygiene and adequate hydration.
14. Assess bowel elimination patterns/instruct about importance of not straining at stool and prescribed measures to treat or avoid constipation (e.g., stool softeners/laxatives, increased dietary fiber, adequate hydration)/evaluate effectiveness of bowel regimen.
15. Observe/instruct about importance of wearing Medic Alert bracelet with information on medical condition and anticoagulant medication.
16. Assess and evaluate alterations in functional skills, self-care deficits/refer to rehabilitative services as ordered to instruct in prescribed graded

cardiac exercise program and energy conservation techniques.

17. Assess/instruct how to summon help in an emergency situation (e.g., dialing 911).
18. Assess anxiety and apprehension associated with altered body image and changes in life-style/

encourage to verbalize concerns about sexual activity to condition/refer to social services to assist with adjustment to illness and provide information regarding community services for assistance with cardiac rehabilitation (e.g., American Heart Association; Smokenders; counseling services).

Legal Glossary

Affidavit. A written statement that is taken under oath

Appeal. A petition to a higher court to review and retry the legal issues and correct or reverse a judgment or decision by a lower court

Appellant. A party who appeals the decision of a lower court to a court of higher jurisdiction

Appellee. The party against whom an appeal to a higher court is taken

Complaint. The first pleading on the part of the plaintiff in a civil action

Civil law. The division of American law that does not deal with crimes

Consent. Voluntary agreement by a competent person to make a choice to allow someone else to do something

Contract. An agreement between two or more persons to do or to refrain from doing something. May be an *express* contract based on declarations either orally or in writing, or an *implied* contract implied by law from the circumstances surrounding a transaction

Defamation. Injury to a person's reputation or character by willful and malicious statements to a third person. *Libel* is by use of written words, *slander* by use of spoken words

Defendant. The person against whom a lawsuit is initiated. Defends himself or herself against allegations by the plaintiff, who seeks legal redress

Damages. A monetary sum or compensation awarded by the court or jury for the loss or harm suffered by the plaintiff

Deposition. Testimony of a witness taken in writing under oath in answer to oral or written questions. Usually used in pretrial phase to prepare for litigation. A person who is being deposed is called a deponent

Due process. A legal concept requiring that legal proceedings or those of a legal nature will be conducted with rules and principles that protect an individual's rights

Comparative negligence. A defense theory in negligence cases where the degree of negligence by the plaintiff is compared to that of the defendant and apportioned accordingly for the purpose of money damages. Used by a majority of states instead of contributory negligence

Contributory negligence. A defense theory in negligence cases based on the idea that the injured party contributed to his own negligence and thus should be barred from recovering any money damages

Evidence. Anything offered to prove or disprove a claim or fact in a legal proceeding. May include documents, objects, testimony of witnesses, or other records

Corporate negligence. Liability of an institution for its failure to use reasonable care in conducting its business

Indemnify. The process of repaying a party for losses brought on when the obligation to repay exists under a contractual provision

Inference. A conclusion reached by the jury from the facts proved

Interrogatories. Written questions about the case submitted to a party by another party that are answered under oath. Part of the pretrial discovery process, but may be used later as evidence

Issue. A single and material point resulting from the allegations of the parties in the lawsuit

Judgment. The decision of the law as given by the court after the legal proceedings

Litigation. A trial in a court for the purpose of establishing rights and duties between parties in a lawsuit

Liability. A legally recognized responsibility one is bound to perform. In negligence law, it is legal responsibility for the loss of another person for one's failure to act, or failure to act appropriately

Liability insurance. A contract to have someone else (the insurer) pay for any loss or liability on the part of the insured in exchange for the payment of premiums. *Occurrence basis policy* covers incidents occurring at the time when premiums were paid. *Claims-made basis policy* covers only if in effect when claim is made (i.e., it is not retroactive to the time of an earlier incident)

Negligence. The failure to use that degree of care equal to a reasonably prudent or careful person acting under the same or similar circumstances. This could involve commission of an act or failure to carry out an act by omission

Plaintiff. The person who initiates the lawsuit against the defendant and seeks legal redress, usually in the form of money damages

Precedent. A ruled case or court decision used as an example of authority for a similar case or one which raises similar issues

Release. A written contract for which some claim or interest in something is surrendered to another person. An example is a release by a client to disclose information to an insurer

Respondent superior. Means "let the master answer." The employer (master) answers for the wrongful acts or negligence of the employee (servant) when acting within the scope of his or her employment

Risk management. A system of identifying potential liability exposure to prevent financial loss. A business concept that identifies and evaluates the probability of financial loss in order to prevent its occurrence

Standard of care. In negligence law, that degree of care and skill that a reasonably prudent person should exercise. In malpractice cases or professional negligence, that degree of skill, care, and knowledge exercised by members of the same discipline

Statute. An act of the legislature declaring, prohibiting, or commanding something. For example, a state nurse practice act is a statute regulating the practice of nurses in a particular state

Statute of limitations. The statutory time limit that a plaintiff has to file a lawsuit. Exceptions include an extension for the time it would reasonably take to "discover" a wrong or a longer time extension if the plaintiff is a minor

Subpoena. An order by the court for a person to appear at a certain time and place to testify on a matter. A *subpoena duces tecum* commands a witness to produce certain documents in his or her possession

Summons. A legal document called a writ, which directs the sheriff or other officer to notify a person that an action (lawsuit) has been started against him or her. Requires the named party or parties (defendants) to appear on a certain day to answer the complaint against them

Tort. A legal wrong committed against a person or the property of another for which the law gives a civil remedy. Exists independent of a contract

Vicarious liability. Liability of a corporation or organization for the negligence of its employees. Based on the idea that the employer receives the benefits of the employees' acts and, therefore, should also be responsible for the burdens of the employees' acts. Employer is in a position to control or supervise the acts of the employee

Drugs and Solutions Most Commonly Used in Home Care

I. ANTIBIOTICS
Acyclovir (Zovirax)
Amphotericin B (Fungizone)
Amikacin
Ampicillin (Omnipen-N,
   Totacillin-N, Polycillin-N)
Azlocillin (Azlin)
Carbenicillin (Geopen, Pyopen)
Cefamandole (Mandol)
Cefazolin (Ancef, Kefzol)
Cefonicid (Monocid)
Cefoperazone (Cefobid)
Ceforanide (Precef)
Cefotaxime (Claforan)
Cefoxitin (Mefoxin)
Ceftizoxime (Cefizox)
Cefuroxime (Zinacef)
Cephalothin (Keflin Neutral)
Cephapirin (Cefadyl)
Chloramphenicol (Chloromycetin)
Clindamycin (Cleocin)
Cyclosporine (Sandimmune)
Erythromycin (Erythrocin)
Gentamicin (Garamycin)
Methicillin (Staphcillin, Celbenin)
Metronidazole (Metro IV)
Mezlocillin (Mezlin)
Miconazole (Monistat)
Moxalactum (Moxam)
Nafcillin (Unipen)
Netilmicin (Netromycin)
Oxacillin (Prostaphlin)
Penicillin G. Potassium
Piperacillin (Pipracil)
Ticarcillin (Ticar)
Tobramycin (Nebcin)
Vancomycin (Vancocin)

II. CHEMOTHERAPEUTICS
Dacarbazine (DTIC)
Dactinomycin (Actinomycin D)
Daunomycin (Cerubidine)
Doxorubicin (Adriamycin)
Mithramycin (Mithracin)
Mitomycin C (Mytamycin)
Estramustine Phosphate (Estracyte)
Vinblastine (Velban)
Vincristine (Oncovin)
Carmustine (BCNU)
Cisplatin (Platinol)
Asparaginase (Elspar)
Etoposide (VP-16, VePesid)
Streptozocin (Zanosar)
Teniposide I+ (VM-26)
Mitoguazone I+ (Methyl-GAG)
Bleomycin (Blenoxane)
Fluorouracil (5-FU)
Cyclophosphamide (Cytoxan)
Cytarabine (ARA-C)
Floxuridine (FUDR)
Methotrexate
Thiotepa

III. NARCOTICS (PAIN MANAGEMENT)
Morphine
Dilaudid
Narcan (Narcotic antagonist)

IV. SOLUTIONS
A. TPN
   Lipids
   Solutions D_5W, NS, Ringer's lactate, $D_5\frac{1}{2}$ NS
B. Additives
   KCl
   Vitamins

V. OTHER
Lasix
Insulin
Dilantin
Heparin
Mannitol
Solu-Medrol
$D_{50}W$

From Med-Center Home Health Care, Danbury, CT, with permission.

Patient Emergency Phone List

Patient Name _____ Phone # _____
Address _____
Home Care Support Services _____
Physician _____ Phone # _____
Equipment Supplier _____ Phone # _____
Hospital _____ Phone # _____
Fire Department _____ Phone # _____
Police Department _____ Phone # _____
Rescue Squad _____ Phone # _____
Ambulance _____ Phone # _____
Electric Company _____ Phone # _____
Phone Company _____ Phone # _____
Emergency Room _____ Phone # _____
Drug Store _____ Phone # _____
Home Care Agency _____ Phone # _____
Primary Home Care Nurse _____ Phone # _____
Pastoral Care _____ Phone # _____
Support Group _____ Phone # _____
Next of Kin _____ Phone # _____
Other _____ Phone # _____
Other _____ Phone # _____

Type of Therapy Receiving and Date (update as changes occur)

Type of Therapy _____ Dose _____ Frequency _____
Equipment Used _____
Equipment Settings _____

Additional Comments _____
_____
_____
_____
_____
_____
_____
_____
_____
_____
_____
_____
_____

From Med-Center Home Health Care, Inc., Danbury, CT, with permission.

Patient Teaching Checklist

Content	Content Reviewed	Return Demonst.	Capable of Self Care	Reliant on Others	Comments
1. Type of Therapy					
2. Drug/solution					
Dose/Schedule					
Label Accuracy					
Storage					
Container Integrity					
Side Effects					
3. Aseptic Technique					
Handwashing					
Prepping Caps/Connects					
Tubing/Cap/Needle Chg					
4. Access Device Maint.					
Type/Name					
Device/Site Inspect					
Site Care/Dsg. Change					
Catheter Clamping					
Maintaining Patency					
Saline/Heparin Flushing					
Feeding Tube Declogging					
5. Drug Preparation					
Premixed Containers					
Compounding					
3:1 Lipid Transfer					
6. Method of Administ.					
Gravity/Pump					
Continuous/Intermit					
Cycle/Taper					
7. Admin. Technique					
Pump Rate/Calibration					
Priming Tubing Filter					
Filling Syringe					
Loading Pump					
Access Device Hookup					
Head Elevation					

Content	Content Reviewed	Return Demonst.	Capable of Self Care	Reliant on Others	Comments
8. Potential Complication					
Pump Alarm					
Trouble Shooting					
Phlebitis/Infiltration					
Clotting/Dislodgement					
Infection/Air Embolis					
Breakage/Cracking					
Electrolyte Imbalance					
Fluid Imbalance					
Glucose Intolerance					
Aspiration					
N/V/D/Cramping					
Other:					
9. Self Monitoring					
Weight/Temperature					
I&O Uringe S/A					
Other:					
10. Supply Handling/Disposal					
Blood/Fluid Precaution					
Chemo/Spill Precaution					
11. Written Instructions to Patient					

(Date and initial each corresponding box and Initial and sign)

Standard High-Tech Care Plans

PLAN OF CARE: HOME IV THERAPY

GOALS:

NAME: _____ TYPE OF SERVICE: _____

DIAGNOSIS(es): 1. Home IV therapy _____ 2. _____

Date	Patient and/or Family Needs and Problems	Unusual Problems	Planned Steps to Meet Needs and Solve Problems	By Whom	Date	Review and Signature
	Hookup and disconnect procedure		Client will be instructed, per procedure, on • Aseptic technique • Spiking IV bag and priming tubing • How to access IV line • Regulation of fluid rate • Heparinization of line • Proper securing with tape The client/caregiver must demonstrate proficiency (to the satisfaction of the PCN) in performing and maintaining therapy to initially enroll and to continue in the home care program.			
	Teaching needs Indications for, and concept of home IV therapy		The client will be taught • The concept of home IV therapy • Indications for home IV therapy (e.g., hydration, antibiotics) • Benefits of home IV therapy Decreased cost Early return to work and ADL Shorter length of hospitalization Decreased incidence of contracting nosocomial infections			
	IV site observation and care		Patient will be instructed to keep site dry (no shower, only sponge baths). Patient will be taught to observe site for redness, streaking, swelling, pain and/or leaking at site, and to notify RN. Patient will be taught the side effects of the specific medication that is being administered			

From C. Winkler RN, BSN, Med-Center Home Health Care, Danbury, CT, with permission.

PLAN OF CARE: HICKMAN CARE

GOALS:

NAME: _____ **TYPE OF SERVICE:** _____

DIAGNOSIS(es): 1. Hickman Care _____ **2.** _____

Date	Patient and/or Family Needs and Problems	Unusual Problems	Planned Steps to Meet Needs and Solve Problems	By Whom	Date	Review and Signature
	Performance of *daily* site care		1. Caregiver will have successfully completed training in Hickman care 2. Caregiver will be able to demonstrate knowledge of what a Hickman catheter is and general safety precautions Hickman catheter care: a. Clean work area with alcohol b. Wash hands with liquid soap for 3 minutes c. Gather supplies and open packages d. Remove old dressing and inspect the site for • Leaking of fluid • Blood or pus • Redness, swelling, or tenderness *Any of the above should be reported immediately to the client's MD or home care nurse. e. Using peroxide-soaked sterile cotton tip applicator, clean exit site following Hickman catheter care instructions, and apply Band-Aid			
	Performance of *daily* heparin flush		1. Immediately following daily site care, wash hands 2. Prepare supplies for flush procedure 3. Flush Hickman catheter with 2.5 cc of heparin following flush procedure instructions			
	Performance of *weekly* cap change		1. Once weekly (or more often if indicated) immediately following site care procedure, and preceding heparin flush, change injection cap following cap change instructions 2. Remove old tape from clamping site and apply new tape. Place tape on a rotating basis, moving from a position close to the skin, outward. Write date on tape.			
	Hickman catheter complications		1. Report immediately any signs and symptoms indicated on signs and symptoms checklist to MD or home care nurse			

PLAN OF CARE: PORT-O-CATH MAINTENANCE

GOALS:

NAME: _____ TYPE OF SERVICE: _____

DIAGNOSIS(es): 1. Port-O-Cath Maintenance _____ 2. _____

Date	Patient and/or Family Needs and Problems	Unusual Problems	Planned Steps to Meet Needs and Solve Problems	By Whom	Date	Review and Signature
	Patient responsibility immediately post-op		Indication for, and explanation of Port-O-Cath will be done by MD and/or nurse A. Initially, gauze will be applied postop (with or without Huber needle inserted in Port-O-Cath, per M.D. discretion). Dressing will be changed after 24 hours and then every 3 days until incision is healed. B. Patient will be instructed to avoid showering for first 10 days, and that when showering to direct spray on his/her back. Dressing must be changed if it becomes wet or loose. C. Patient will be aware of possibility of swelling around site for up to 2 weeks post-op			
	Long-term		A. Patient will be taught to inspect site for leakage of fluid/infiltration/hematoma, redness, streaking, or tenderness along catheter track. B. If patient is to access Port-O-Cath he/she will be taught per agency procedure specifically hookup, disconnection, and heparinization of Port-O-Cath.			

PLAN OF CARE: PORT-O-CATH MAINTENANCE

GOALS:

NAME: _____ TYPE OF SERVICE: _____

DIAGNOSIS(es): 1. Port-O-Cath Maintenance _____ 2. _____

Date	Patient and/or Family Needs and Problems	Unusual Problems	Planned Steps to Meet Needs and Solve Problems	By Whom	Date	Review and Signature
	Accessing line		Using aseptic technique A. Set up sterile field, per procedure B. Using #18g Huber needle and extension tubing, prime with NS, and clamp C. Clean site, per procedure, with Betadine. D. Palpate Port-O-Cath with one hand, locating center E. With other hand, push needle perpendicularly through skin into center of device until needle stops F. Open clamp on extension tubing and infuse solution			
	Long-term therapy		For continuous or long-term therapy A. An air occlusive window dressing will be applied B. The needle and occlusive dressing will be changed by an RN weekly C. Line will be primed, per procedure D. Dressing will be applied, per procedure E. Dressing will be secured with tape to form a window frame, and extension tubing will be secured on top			
	Disconnecting line		Using aseptic technique A. Draw up NS and heparin, per procedure B. Clean connection with three alcohol wipes between extension tubing and cap, or pump tubing C. Inject NS and heparin, per procedure. Close clamp D. Remove dressing E. With Betadine, cleanse site, per procedure F. Place thumb and forefinger of one hand on either side of needle, grip hub and pull upward. With other hand, apply pressure to decrease incidence of hematoma			
	Troubleshooting		A. For spontaneous blood backflow, patient should check connections and tighten, and check pump function B. Leaking: Check connections and tighten. Retape C. Catheter occlusion: Clamp extension tubing and notify MD/PCN. Instruct patient not to flush D. For extravasation: Instruct patient to notify MD/PCN Note needle placement, backflow of blood, catheter disconnection, attempt to aspirate bid. Consider: Cracked or separated catheter from Port-O-Cath E. Withdrawal occlusion: Check needle placement, have patient change position Consider: Thrombosis, cracked or separated catheter Instruct patient to notify MD/PCN with the following signs and symptoms A. Fever greater than 101° B. Swelling, redness, tenderness or discharge at site, or blood backup in tubing C. Swelling and/or pain in area of collarbone, neck, face, or upper arm D. Prominent veins in neck, face, arm, or chest E. Difficulty swallowing F. Sores in mouth, diarrhea, nausea, or vomiting			

PLAN OF CARE: TPN

GOALS:

NAME: _____   TYPE OF SERVICE: _____

DIAGNOSIS(es): 1. TPN _____   2. _____

Date	Patient and/or Family Needs and Problems	Unusual Problems	Planned Steps to Meet Needs and Solve Problems	By Whom	Date	Review and Signature
	Observation/recording and precautions		Need to monitor • Serum Electrolytes - P_{12} weekly • Urine dipsticks for greater than 1+ glycosuria • Weight/nutritional status • Vital signs • Hickman catheter site (See care plan) • Distended veins in neck, arms, hands secondary to central venous thrombosis • Swelling/edema in face, neck, head secondary to infiltration of solution into surrounding tissues			
	Teaching needs: Patient and significant others		• Check temperature (M–W–F), notify nurse of elevation. Check temp. more frequently if patient feels ill • Weight/urine dipstick (M–W–F) and document. Check more frequently if patient feels ill • Importance of balanced diet and adequate elimination • Notify nurse of weight gain or loss more than 2 lbs. • Notify nurse of any of the following symptoms: Excessive cramping, gas accumulation, diarrhea, nausea, vomiting, constipation, large urine output, decrease in appetite, if applicable • Teaching and reinforcement of aseptic handwashing technique and maintaining sterility of IV solution delivery system			

Clinical Flow Sheet

	DATE	DATE	DATE	DATE
Vital Signs				
Intake: Oral 　　　Intravenous 　　　Enteral				
Output: Urine 　　　Stool 　　　Other				
Neurological: (confusion, orientation)				
Respiratory (S.O.B., Rales, Rhonchi)				
Gastrointestinal (N/V/D, constipation)				
Genito-Urinary (color, characteristics)				
Hematological (bleeding, bruising)				
Cardiac (palpitations, edema, syncope, heart sounds)				
Musculo-Skeletal (pain, decreased R.O.M.)				
Medication Reactions (describe relative to prescribed medications)				
Intravenous: 　Catheter Site: 　(appearance, dressing change) 　Restart/Re-access 　Flow/Troubleshooting				
Enteral: (describe flow & tolerance) Placement checked				
Lab tests drawn				
Teaching topics (describe topic and patient reaction)				
See Care Plan (yes/no)				
See Physician Orders (yes/no)				
See Narrative note (yes/no)				
Signature				

Laboratory Flow Sheet

PATIENT: _____   RECORD NUMBER: _____
            LAB: _____

LAB VALUES (Adult values)

DATE									
CHEMISTRY:									
Sodium(135-148mE/L)									
Potassium(3.5-5.3mEq/L)									
Chloride(95-100mEq/L)									
Bicarb(24mEq/L)									
Co2(24-30mEq/L)									
BUN (10-20mg/dl)									
Creat(0.7-1.5 mg/dl)									
Glucose(70-125mg/dl)									
Calcium(8.5-10.7mg/dl)									
Ionized Ca(3.8-4.5 mg/dl)									
Magnesium(1.8-2.5mEq/L)									
Phosphorus(2.5-4.5mg/dl)									
Uric Acid(3-8.5mg/dl)									
Total Protein(6-8.5g/dl)									
Albumin(3.5-5.5g/dl)									
Triglycerides(20-190mg/dl)									
Cholesterol(150-300 mg/dl)									
Iron(50-150ug/dl)									
TIBC(250-410ug/dl)%sat									
LIVER FUNCTION TESTS:									
LDH(0-250 U/ml)									
SGOT/SGPT (0-50 U/ml)									
Alk Phos (20-140 IU/L)									
HEMOTOLOGY:									
RBC(4.2-5.4 mil/cu mm)									
WBC(4-10,800/cu mm)									
Platelets(130-140/cu mm)									
Hgb(14-17 g/dl)									
Hct(43-51%)									
MCV(83.6-103.6/cu micron)									
MCH(27-31 pg)									

PATIENT: _____   **RECORD NUMBER:** _____

LAB: _____

LAB VALUES (Adult values) (Cont.)

MCHC(32-36%)									
PT/PTT									
Trace Elements									
Drug: Peak									
Trough									
Other:									

Generic Pediatric Home Care Plan for Families with an Ill Child

GENERAL PSYCHOSOCIAL ISSUES FOR FAMILIES

Assessment

Overall, ongoing observation of home environment and family interaction:

- Is it nurturing and supportive to the ill child?
- Is parental anxiety interfering with parent–child bonding.
- Are interactions between parents positive and supportive?
- Are parents able to communicate appropriately with health professionals?
- How are siblings reacting and adjusting?
- Are parents feeling isolated and exhausted from the ongoing responsibilities of home care?

Nursing Interventions

1. Promote parents' self-esteem and confidence by commending their accomplishments with the child.

2. Act as a role model in meeting the ill child's and sibling's physical, developmental, and emotional needs.
3. Allow parents the time and opportunity to discuss their lives and feelings.
4. Offer emotional support without encouraging dependency.
5. Identify a case manager (usually the primary home care nurse) and clearly define what needs to be communicated.
6. Suggest appropriate support groups, organizations, or agencies to assist with financial, social, or mental health needs.
7. Assist parents in problem solving by identifying respite programs, arranging for private duty nursing, or identifying friends/family who could offer assistance.

(See Specific Care Plans, next four pages)

Generic Home Care Plan for the Child Receiving IV Therapy

Assessment

Physical	Psychosocial	Developmental
1. State the child's diagnosis and its associated high-tech management (e.g., osteomyelitis of right tibia requiring 6 weeks IV antibiotic treatment)	1. Describe child's and family's reaction to venipuncture and IV procedures	1. Describe the child's behavior reactions to IV therapy and if appropriate for developmental stage
2. Describe pertinent health history	2. Observe general parenting skills and parental support	2. Note if child is able to participate in regular school program or requires home tutoring
3. Record baseline vital signs cardiopulmonary, HEENT, GI, GU, neuro, musculoskeletal, and integumentary status		
4. Describe functional disabilities relating to play or ADLs		
5 Describe location of IV site and if peripheral or central		
6 State how often peripheral IV site dressing or central IV dressing to be changed		

Nursing Interventions

Equipment	Teaching	Safety Checklist
1 List all types of equipment necessary. The following is a comprehensive list: • IV solution(s) • IV pump • IV needles (angiocath or butterfly) • Syringes and needles • Medications • Arm board • Tubex • Transparent dressing (e.g., Tegarderm, Opsite, Duoderm) • Heparin solution • Saline • Heparin lock adaptor • Alcohol and Betadine swabs • Injection cap • Padded clamp • Needle disposal container • Hydrogen peroxide • Central line catheter repair kit	1 Review child's diagnosis and reasons for IV and medications 2. Signs of IV complications: infiltration, infection 3. Demonstrate and redemonstrate IV setup procedure using appropriate sterile technique 4. Demonstrate and redemonstrate use of equipment 5. Who and when to call in event of complications or equipment malfunction	1. Are there adequate trained caregivers? 2. Are equipment and suppliers child proofed or in a safe location? 3. Is there a backup plan if peripheral IV cannot be started at home?

Generic Home Care Plan for the Child with a Respiratory Problem
(apnea monitor, oxygen, tracheostomy, ventilator)

Assessment

Physical

1. State the child's diagnosis and its associated high-tech management (e.g., tracheal stenosis requiring tracheostomy, oxygen, and apnea monitor)
2. Describe pertinent health history
3. Record baseline weight, height, head circumference, vital signs, breath sounds, retractions, color, nasal flaring
4. Describe type, amount of feedings, position for feedings, special bottles, nipples, spoons
5. Describe functional disabilities relating to play or ADLs
6. Describe sleep/wake patterns

Psychosocial

Observe and record:
1. Parenting skills
2. Parent–child bonding
3. Siblings' response to ill child
4. Parent sharing and support

Developmental

1. Observe child's developmental stage in relation to actual age (e.g., no verbal skills for 3-year-old)
2. Describe child's limitations and potential (e.g., tires quickly with motor activity but has good muscle tone)
3. Note infant stimulation programs or school programs child may be involved in or referred to

Nursing Interventions

Equipment

1. List all types of equipment necessary. The following is a comprehensive list:
   - Ventilator
   - Oxygen source
   - Oxygen tent
   - Nasal cannula
   - Trach mask
   - Extra tubing
   - Humidity source
   - Ambu bag
   - Sterile water or saline
   - Suction machine and catheters
   - Monitor leads and electrode pads
   - Monitor belt
   - Battery pack

Teaching

1. Signs of respiratory distress specific to this child
2. How to respond to alarms
3. Infant/child CPR
4. Review plan in event of emergency
5. Suctioning and chest physiotherapy
6. Review child's diagnosis and reasons for equipment
7. Demonstration with redemonstration on use and cleaning of equipment
8. Review oxygen monitor ventilator settings
9. Medications: actions, side effects, and contraindications

Safety Checklist

1. Are there adequately trained caregivers?
2. Can alarms be heard from all locations?
3. Are emergency numbers posted?
4. Are equipment and medications child proofed or in a safe location?
5. Are equipment manuals available?
6. Are no sources of combustion present?
7. Is a fire extinguisher available?
8. Is there a source of power in event of blackout?

Generic Home Care Plan for the Child with a Gastrointestinal/Nutritional Problem (feeding tubes, colostomies, feeding pumps)

Assessment

Physical

1. State the child's diagnosis and its associated high-tech management (e.g., gastroesophogeal reflux requiring duodenal tube feedings and gastrostomy tube placement)
2. Describe pertinent health history
3. Record baseline weight, height, head circumference, growth percentiles, bowel function/sounds, vomiting, oral feedings, skin around stoma
4. Describe type, amount, rate of feedings
5. Describe functional disabilities relating to play or ADLs
6. Describe sleep/wake pattern in relation to feedings

Psychosocial

Observe and record:
1. Parenting skills
2. Parent–child bonding
3. Siblings' response to altered feeding procedure
4. Parent sharing and support

Developmental

1. Observe child's developmental stage in relation to actual age
2. Describe child's limitations and potential (e.g., child will suck on pacifier but refuses to swallow)
3. Note infant stimulation or school programs child may be involved in or referred to

Nursing Interventions

Equipment

1. List all types necessary. The following is a comprehensive list:
   - Nasogastric tubes
   - Gastrostomy tube
   - Stethescope
   - Syringes
   - Feeding pump & bags
   - Liquid food
   - Colostomy bags
   - Stoma protectant
   - Catheter adapters

Teaching

1. Review child's diagnosis and reasons for equipment
2. Signs of feeding intolerance
3. Demonstration with redemonstration on use and cleaning of equipment
4. Skin care and/or dressing changes for stoma
5. Medications: actions, side effects, administration

Safety Checklist

1. Are there adequately trained caregivers?
2. Are equipment and medications child proofed and in a safe location?
3. Are equipment manuals available?
4. Is there a backup method of feeding in the event of pump malfunction?

Generic Home Care Plan for the Infant Receiving Home Phototherapy

Assessment

Physical

1. State the infant's diagnosis and its associated high-tech management (e.g., hyperbilirubinemia requiring phototherapy)
2. Describe pertinent health history
3. Record baseline vital signs, weight, general appearance, skin, hydration status, elimination patterns
4. Sleep/wake patterns in relation to feedings

Psychosocial

1. Parenting skills
2. Parent–child bonding
3. Siblings' response
4. Parent sharing and support

Developmental

1. Infant's behavioral response to phototherapy (lethargy, irritability, quiet, alert, etc.)
2. Is infant held and touched when away from lights for feedings?

Nursing Interventions

Equipment

1. List all types of equipment necessary. The following is a comprehensive list:
   • Eye patches
   • Thermometers

Teaching

1. Review diagnosis and reasons for equipment
2. Demonstration and redemonstration of axillary temperature procedure and frequency
3. Turn infant every 2–3 hours
4. Demonstration and redemonstration of application and positioning of eye patches
5. Documentation procedure for feedings, elimination, temperature, and position changes
6. Guidelines for when to call health professionals
7. Necessity for regular heel-stick bilirubin levels

Safety Checklist

1. Are caregivers available to observe the infant at all times?
2. Are equipment and supplies out of reach of siblings?

Pediatric Home Care Resource List

American Cancer Society
777 Third Avenue
New York, NY 10017
1-800-4-CANCER

American Lung Assoc.
1740 Broadway
New York, NY 10019
1-(212)245-8000

Association for the Care
of Children's Health (ACCH)
3615 Wisconsin Avenue, NW
Washington, DC 20016
1-(202)244-1801

Candlelighters Childhood
Cancer Foundation
2025 I Street, NW #1011
Washington, DC 20006
1-(202)659-5136

Children's Hospice
International
501 Slater's Lane #207
Alexandria, VA 22314
1-(804)684-0330

Cystic Fibrosis Foundation
6000 Executive Boulevard #309
Rockville, MD 20852
1-800-344-4823

Families Together
Box 926
Lawrence, KS 66044
1-(913)841-7241

Leukemia Society of America
733 Third Avenue, 14th Floor
New York, NY 10017
1-(212)679-1939

Muscular Dystrophy Association
of America
810 Seventh Avenue
New York, NY 10019
1-(212)586-0808

National Easter Seal Society
2023 West Ogden Avenue
Chicago, IL 60612
1-(312)243-8400

National Information Center for
Handicapped Children and Youth
Box 1492
Washington, DC 20013
1-(202)522-3332

Parents Helping Parents, Inc.
47 Maro Drive
San Jose, CA 95127
1-(408)224-4748

Parents of Premature and High
Risk Infants International, Inc.
33 West 42 Street, Suite 1227
New York, NY 10036
1-(212)840-1259

Sick Kids Need Involved People (SKIP)
216 Newport Drive
Saverna Park, MD 21146
1-(202)261-2602

United Cerebral Palsy Association, Inc.
66 East 34th Street
New York, NY 10010
1-(212)481-6300

Medicare Documentation Hints

- Medicare services acutely ill patients in an unstable condition. Make sure the diagnosis reflects an acute illness. For example, instead of writing diabetes mellitus × 10 years, write uncontrolled diabetes × 15 days.

- Avoid using words such as "stable or status quo" in any of the documentation.

- The patient must be homebound. Homebound status should be clearly documented in the chart. If the client's diagnosis is one which may not make the client homebound, explain why this particular client is unable to leave his home.

- All home care services must be provided under a plan of care signed by the physician. Doctors orders consist of the 485-486. These orders must be renewed every 60 days. All services should be reflected in the M.D. orders.

- Skilled services include nursing, physical therapy and speech therapy. Other services including occupational therapy, medical social worker and home health aide are covered by Medicare only when a skilled service involved with the plan of care.

- Medicare defines "skilled" based on the inherent complexity of the service, condition of the patient, and accepted standards of practice. Clearly describe the skilled service provided on each home visit. The skilled service should be consistent with the diagnosis of the client.

- Document all teaching to client and significant other. Be careful to avoid words such as "reinforced or reinstructed". Medicare will not pay for reinforcement of teaching. Use words and phrases such as "instructed, instructed again, return demonstration provided by client".

- Document the condition of the client without subjective interpretation. For example, avoid saying the wound is healing. Instead, write the wound is 1″ long by ½″ wide by ¼″ deep.

- Whenever possible, quantify the client's condition Measure and document all wounds, swelling, edema of extremities, or ascites.

- Document Home Health Aide supervision every two weeks. Case conferences with other services (i.e., P.T., O.T., M.S.W.) involved in the plan of care must be documented in the chart

Index

Page numbers followed by *t* refer to tables. Page numbers followed by *f* refer to figures.

Page numbers followed by *t* refer to tables. Page numbers followed by *f* refer to figures.

Page numbers followed by *t* refer to tables. Page numbers followed by *f* refer to figures.

Page numbers followed by t refer to tables. Page numbers followed by f refer to figures.

NOTES

NOTES

NOTES